Research on Language and Social Interaction

VOLUME 35, NUMBER 2 — 2002

Table of Contents

Most Commonly Used Transcription Symbols

.	(period) Falling intonation.
?	(question mark) Rising intonation.
,	(comma) Continuing intonation.
-	(hyphen) Marks an abrupt cut-off.
::	(colon(s)) Prolonging of sound.
ne<u>v</u>er	(underlining) Stressed syllable or word.
WORD	(all caps) Loud speech.
°word°	(degree symbols) Quiet speech.
>word<	(more than & less than) Quicker speech.
<word>	(less than & more than) Slowed speech.
hh	(series of h's) Aspiration or laughter.
.hh	(h's preceded by dot) Inhalation.
[ ]	(brackets) Simultaneous or overlapping speech.
=	(equals sign) Contiguous utterances.
(2.4)	(number in parentheses) Length of a silence.
(.)	(period in parentheses) Micro-pause, 2/10 second or less.
( )	(empty parentheses) Non-transcribable segment of talk.
(word)	(word or phrase in parentheses) Transcriptionist doubt.
((gazing toward the ceiling))	(double parentheses) Description of non-speech activity.

Research on Language and Social Interaction, 35(2), 115–137
Copyright © 2002, Lawrence Erlbaum Associates, Inc.

Discourse, Expertise, and the Management of Risk in Health Care Settings

Christopher N. Candlin
Center for English Language Education and Communication Research
City University of Hong Kong

Sally Candlin
Department of Nursing, Family, and Community Health
University of Western Sydney, New South Wales

This special issue identifies three interrelated constructs—discourse, expertise, and the definition and management of risk—located in various health care sites: genetic counseling, nursing, and medical practice. The articles highlight the relation between the management of risk situations and the nature of expertise displayed or achieved by practitioners and their patients or clients. Professional expertise is differentiated and multifaceted, concerning not only the exercise of discipline-specific professional practices and behaviors but also intimately related to the management of discoursal practices. The articles suggest that health care outcomes can be related closely to the quality of the discoursal encounters between professional practitioners and their patients or clients, among professional practitioners themselves, or both. The research we present evidences differentiated goals and outcomes from a range of professional encounters. It focuses especially on the resource of discoursal strategies drawn on in the achievement of discoursal and professional goals by both professional and lay participants.

Correspondence concerning this article should be sent to Christopher N. Candlin, Center for English Language Education and Communication Research, City University of Hong Kong, Tat Chee Avenue, Kowloon, Hong Kong. E-mail: ccandlin@pacific.net.hk

This special issue of *Research on Language and Social Interaction* contains four empirical articles in which authors discuss issues emerging from the display of expertise in the domain of health care as it is mediated through discourse, particularly in the context of the management of risk. The articles draw on distinctive but interrelated research traditions, although the methodologies of all are concerned with the analysis of naturally occurring interaction. Three of the articles (S. Candlin; Sarangi & Clarke; and Linell, Adelswärd, Sachs, Bredmar, & Lindstedt) focus on qualitative analysis, whereas the fourth by Peräkylä links qualitative with quantitative analysis. All indicate the importance of including reference to institutional factors in their explanations of data and some—especially the first three—to broader sociological factors in the social formation. All are committed to the local and contextualized analysis of particular encounters, either focusing on a particular site and specialism, or usefully making comparisons across different sites and specialisms within primary health care and with different orders of professional and types of patient or client. All adopt a position that, despite situationally and individually motivated variation, the discursive expression of expertise is to different extents a coparticipative endeavor of all involved. Finally, all contributors have direct and firsthand experience of the sites in question through their research and professional commitment to the study of reflective practice in health care communication. Some of the authors are doubly qualified and experienced in health care and discourse analysis, thus underpinning the close association between expert practitioner and analyst that this special issue seeks in part to promote.

CONCEPTUALIZING RISK AND EXPERTISE IN THE DISCOURSE OF HEALTH PROFESSIONALS

In correlating the discourse of professional activity with the conceptualizing of professional expertise in the context of risk management in health care, four issues suggest themselves:

1. What synergy is there between discourse and professional expertise?
2. What constitutes expert activity in health care?

3. How is expertise to be contextualized and how is it realized in discourse?
4. How is risk managed in health care settings?

WHAT SYNERGY IS THERE BETWEEN
DISCOURSE AND PROFESSIONAL EXPERTISE?

Communicative ability understood as the strategic deployment of discursive resources is explicitly signaled as a marker of expert behavior in a wide range of professional activities (and increasingly across many nonprofessional workplaces). The signaling of this linkage has been addressed directly by references to communicative ability in the competency statements of such professions, often couched in terms of being a marker of stages toward being expert, as in nursing (S. Candlin, 1997) and a variety of other fields. In this context, in some domains such as speech pathology, some publications—as, for example, Kovarsky, Duchan, and Maxwell (1999)—have problematized the way the link between communicative and professional expertise has been typically reduced to simple lists of desirable communicative features. These authors, advocate, in contrast, the display of evidence for expertise to be drawn from a more contextualized and differentiated accounting of communicative behaviors in practice. More generally, for example in the industrial training field, attempts have been made (see Cheetham & Chivers, 1998) to harmonize competency and knowledge-driven approaches to the defining of expertise with Schön's (1983, 1987) classic advocacy of the study of professionals' reflective practice: what he termed *artistry* or *knowing in action*. Such harmonization identifies communicative ability as a key element in the determination of expert behavior but insists on evidence from detailed ethnographic accounts of such expertise in action. From the perspective of discourse and conversational analysis, researchers concerned with professional–client interaction, or workplace communication more generally, for their part frequently introduce the concept of *expertise* or *expert behavior* in their accounts of talk and writing—in particularly focused encounters— and assert a linkage between discursive ability and expertise. As one example, such ability is identified as a fundamental resource in health care practice in terms of creating the contexts within which professional care-givers and patients can make their intentions known as a preliminary toward problem identification, exploration, and treatment. In some medical and health care specialisms, as in psychiatry and psychotherapy—or, as we indicated previously, in disciplines like speech pathology—the display of communicative ability by the professional is central to the profession's self-definition, not merely some necessary adjunct.

Much less common, however, from either perspective is the attempt by both bodies of experts to align discourse analytical insights with insights into the nature of professional work, with the aim of exploring the nature both of professional expertise and how it may be displayed in discourse and, more important, what the synergies between them might be. It is this question that the authors of the articles in this special issue seek to address.

A number of issues immediately arise in asserting such synergy. First, how is expertise to be defined in context—generally, cross sectorally within a professional field, or discipline specifically—and in relation to which critical issues confronting the professional field and discipline in question? Second, how is discursive competence to be defined (again, cross sectorally, or discipline specifically and sector specifically, and in relation to which core issues)? From this, third, what are the features of this discursive competence for consideration as candidates for the identification of expertise, which may contribute in various ways to its enhancement, and how are both calibrated and evaluated?

The articles in this special issue are in part aimed at addressing these questions. They do so in the professional field of health care; within this, in the specialism of genetic counseling; and in a range of other specialist contexts within primary health care, for example in patient assessment in nursing, in midwifery, and in doctor–patient interaction in general practice. All of the authors have significant experience in collaborative work either as discourse analysts, health care professionals, or both. Three of the four articles in this issue (S. Candlin; Linell et al.; Sarangi & Clarke) direct their analyses to the critical issue of how risk is negotiated and managed in different settings of health care practice, whereas that of Peräkylä provides a necessary backdrop to such negotiation by examining how doctors' expertise in the appraisal and calculation of risk in diagnosis is not just a matter of the exercise of authority but one of maintaining a specific balance between authority and accountability vis-à-vis their patients.

WHAT CONSTITUTES EXPERT
ACTIVITY IN HEALTH CARE?

In her article for this special issue, S. Candlin draws on Benner's (1984) definition of expert performance in relation to the profession of nursing:

> The expert performer [is one] who no longer relies on analytic principle (rules, guidelines, maxims). The expert nurse, with an enormous background of experience, now has an intuitive grasp of each situation and zeroes in on the accurate region of the problem without wasteful consideration of a large range of alternative diagnoses and solutions. (pp. 31–32)

This definition itself forms part of an analysis of a proposed five-stage development of the expert nurse, captured explicitly in the title of Benner's (1984) book, *From Novice to Expert: Excellence and Power in Clinical Nursing Practice.*

Although such a definition is sector specific, its ultimate source was the work of Dreyfuss and Dreyfuss (1980), who examined the development of skills among airline pilots. Its potential generalizability, therefore, lies in its identifying a number of attributes of expertise, each of which figures in the articles of this special issue. Such attributes can be identified in terms of a resource of institutional *knowledge* and professional *experience* (Sarangi & Roberts, 1999b) and the links between them as necessary underpinnings of the exercise of professional *judgment.* As Cicourel (1992) evidenced in the field of medical diagnosis, such judgment is never abstracted from context, both local and more broadly conceived. In our view, it is always situated against some specific *cost–benefit analysis,* and realized through some event- and person-sensitive *performance.*

One of the concerns for this special issue is how such expert attributes are displayed through particular discursive choices, and whether, even within as broad a professional field as health care, interdisciplinary comparisons of expert behavior are possible. As it happens, health care offers a particularly good site for the discussion of the nature of expertise. In contemporary sociological and social theoretical writing it serves as a classic exemplar of the blurring of boundaries in late modernity and the consequent contestation between professional and lay spheres. As expert knowledge becomes pluralized and disseminated, its underlying beliefs altered, and its traditional asymmetrical distributions of power recast, health care serves as a key site where professionals typically may struggle to reclaim institutionally backed authority as a means of reiterating their institutionally sanctioned expert roles (Giddens, 1990, 1991). Also, contrasts between expert knowledge and lay knowledge—seen as contrasts between what Sarangi and Clarke (2002) call "in-depth mastery of a field of knowledge" versus nonspecific, "typical" knowledge—are themselves breaking down in the field of health care as the focus of authority shifts more to a partnership model of health care provider and patient or client. Such a partnership or "therapeutic alliance" is now expressly advocated by professional bodies (see Royal Pharmaceutical Society of Great Britain, 1997), bringing profound consequences for the practice of health care professionals. As C. N. Candlin, Moore, and Plum (1998) pointed out in a discussion of the relationships in HIV–AIDS health care between patients' involvement in determining treatment regimes and their adherence to them, this move from a *compliance* metaphor to one of *concordance* explicitly expands the partnership construct to that of some mutually entered-into contract. In the field of nursing, S. Candlin (2000) spoke of a "new dynamics" in the relationship between nurses and patients occasioned by such a shift. Central to such a partnership would appear to be what Parks (1998) was identifying when she indicated that patient autonomy is a core concern of almost all treatments of health care ethics, where autonomy is seen as one aspect of partnership, implying the extending to others of the authority to make meaningful and significant life choices. As one example, Haley, Clair, and Saulsberry (1991) referred to optimal medical care as being a judicious mix of doctor-provided and patient-provided information, a display of sensitivity to caregiver and patient concerns, and an attenuation of the degree of doctor dominance over the interaction. Such factors are addressed by Linell et al. and Peräkylä in this issue.

One of the purposes of this special issue, however, is to highlight other grounds for this focus on partnership beyond those moral or ethical issues concerning patients' rights over their bodies and their health. Legal issues concerning malpractice and litigation have become increasingly central, as Sarangi and Clarke (2002) allude to in their article, often in the context of the degree of mutuality established between professional explanation and patient understanding and acceptance, as also evidenced in the article by Peräkylä (2002). The significance of such a partnership for the elicitation by the professional of crucial information from the patient for the management of care is a central theme of S. Candlin's (2002) article and is essential to the discussion in Linell et al.'s (2002) article of the link between explanation and the understanding of risk.

Significant questions thus attend such a call for partnership and are explicitly raised or inhere in this special issue. One such question, and in relation to the implicit assertion of some cocontractual status between the partners, concerns the problematic focus on the individuality of the partnership or contract. With whom is the contract? How able are the partners, especially patients, to enter freely and equally into such a relationship? How clear can the terms and goals of the partnership be made? As Parks (1998) indicated, choices made by a patient remain unproblematic only as long as she or he is not constrained by external factors such as lack of information or lack of options, or is not placed in a coercive situation inhibiting the free exercise of choice. Because this is almost always axiomatically the case, in Parks's view and that of other feminist commentators such as Sherwin (1992), the social context of the partnership can never be irrelevant to the matter of achieving equality in this contractual relationship. This is not only a matter of a gendered perspective on the health care encounter. It has to be pervasive. Issues of difference in relation to class, ethnicity, race, value systems, schemata, and prior knowledge can all lead to inequalities, which in turn can compromise this supposed free contractual status. Any graded staging toward expertise (Benner, 1984) thus takes on an added enculturation dimension in which an important feature of acquired situation-specific competence needs to be set within a much broader historical and social structural perspective. Part of such a perspective is this difficulty of clearly delineating between expert and lay knowledge, as patients (as well as health care professionals) are increasingly enabled to tap into professional and institutional knowledge, for example through health care Web sites and support groups (see Sarangi & Clarke, 2002). In many health care sites and domains the quasi-professional knowledge and experience of the patient may, at moments and in relation to particular terms and experiences, elevate the patient to temporary expert status and change the balance of expertise between the professional and the lay party. This theme is an explicit focus of a recent study of patients with HIV–AIDS interacting with doctors (Moore, Candlin, & Plum, 2001). Sarangi (1998) further elaborated on this mingling of expertise by pointing out not only that the boundaries of expertise are blurred interprofessionally, intraprofessionally, and between professional and client, but also that we may need to further distinguish among what he referred to as "proto-professionals, professional clients and lay clients" (p. 303) and take note, in particular, of the "appropriation of expert voices by professional clients" (p. 304). The detailed accounts of professional–patient interaction in this special issue provide further evidence of such co-construction and the consequent redrawing of the boundaries of expertise.

HOW IS EXPERTISE TO BE CONTEXTUALIZED AND HOW IS IT REALIZED IN DISCOURSE?

Calls for expertise to be linked to discursive action require expertise to be localized and contextualized. The characteristics of such expertise need to be displayed systematically as products of the interactants' orientations to specific features of the interaction. Such a position is routine to all conversational and discourse analytical studies. The issue, of course, remains as to what is meant by "the specific features of the interaction." At one level, this relates to disciplinary specific, intraprofessional, and institutionally sanctioned behaviors: as, for example, within a particular specialism or among different branches of health care, or, more interprofessionally, as between the institutional and professional practices of lawyers and doctors. Expertise is multifaceted and needs to be narrowly located. At the same time, an important matter before the authors in this special issue was that of determining whether, and to what extent, the explanation of specific features of the interaction should be linked to broader, macrostructures of the social formation (Coupland, Sarangi, & Candlin, 2001; Fairclough, 1992; Giddens, 1979). If so, it remains to indicate how, methodologically, these macrostructures can be shown to impinge on the locally managed contexts of interaction (Hak, 1999; Hilbert, 1990) through the evidence provided from the discursive and professional behaviors of participants and their accounts.

We could begin by considering Fahy and Smith's (1999) position that interactionist accounts of health care discourse have, in their view, typically concentrated on the inscription of selves and "illness actions" as emergent properties of local, institutional situations and biographical experiences, and from that go on to ask what other factors might be relevant to any explanatory account (Fairclough, 1992). Fahy and Smith were concerned, as was Cicourel (1992), that too close an insistence on the local may mean that powerful models that have a relation to the general issue of the display of expert behavior, and that can be applied across institutional and cultural contexts, may thus be precluded. In their view, there is a need to incorporate into analyses and explanations discussion of those extra-institutional structural conditions that shape the selves of the participants through encounters that reproduce relationships of power. The thrust of their argument is that the shifting identities and roles of professionals and patients in the course of health care interactions make it necessary for analysts to avoid too great a focus on what Lynch and Bogen (1994) termed the *disembodied utterance*. From the latter's cultural studies perspective, they argued for a greater concentration on a Foucaultian analysis directed at explaining the struggles between and among these identities as they are played out in the discourses. This dimension is addressed directly in S. Candlin's article in this issue in which she discusses issues surrounding the distribution of power in the nurse–patient relationship. For Lynch and Bogen, understanding the relation between expertise and its articulation through discourse needs what Deveaux (1994) spoke of when she called for greater reference to socially structured, wider, and more varied human experiences and identities (in terms of race, class, gender inequalities, and life histories) that for her inform particular encounters within the medical institution. What is clear is not just that such factors will impinge on the conduct of the interaction but that the adoption of multiple subject positions by professional practitioners or patients in such institutions in the course of an encounter makes the demands on discursive competence of both parties more difficult, especially in the coconstructive context of that partnership that we referred to earlier. It also makes the attribution and location of expertise more difficult to capture and pin down, given the complex hybridity characteristic of such discourse (Sarangi, 2000; Sarangi & Roberts, 1999a).

One example of this matter of distinct subject positions is contained in Cameron and Williams's (1997) analysis of a non-native English-speaking nurse working in a U.S. psychiatric hospital. Following work by Galanti (1991) and Panagua (1994) into intercultural communication in health care, they argued that expertise on the part of the professional implies not only encouraging the successful management by both parties of various discursive strategies designed to achieve the professional practitioner's and the patient's goals, but also doing so in contexts in which the selection and employment of these strategies is potentially conditioned by the following differences between both parties: (a) different perceptions by both parties of the origins and meanings of illness, (b) different conceptions by both parties of how patients should respond to illness, (c) different roles taken by both parties in the process of responding to illness, and (d) different ways of speaking by both parties about and to illness.

The articles in this special issue underscore the importance of these factors and widen their relevance to the interpretation of culture as institutional membership. Here there is, of course, no need to isolate the nonnative speaker as a particular case. The point is a general one. As M. R. Haug (1994) and S. Candlin (2002) identify, the same could be easily said of native English-speaking health care professionals interacting with older patients and their caregivers.

There are further conditioning factors on the exercise of discursive choice in the construction and realization of expertise in health care, some of which vary considerably across health care systems. The international perspective afforded by the articles, thus, is one of this special issue's strengths. The degree of partnership health care systems encourage is clearly one such factor, as is the extent of the professional's experience. Another is the double challenge that health care practitioners have to meet in conducting encounters in both a professional (therapeutic) and an interpersonal (social) manner, and managing the discursive challenges of both. The administrative framework of health care delivery within which professionals have to operate in a given system is highly relevant, as where within managed care systems boundaries of time and cost are set on the nature and extent of professional practitioner–patient interactions (Warren, Weitz, & Kulis, 1998). As Stivers (1998) evidenced in an analysis of professional–client interaction in a veterinary clinic, the discursive partnership between professional practitioner and client in determining a diagnosis is continually shaped by awareness on the part of both parties of the cost of various treatment and diagnostic testing options. As we suggested earlier, the evaluation of the display of expertise through discourse is subject to cost–benefit analysis.

Mishler's (1984) picture of the expert doctor who acknowledges the patient's life world and who seeks to minimize the distance between herself or himself while allowing patients to present extended accounts of their own feelings with minimum interruptions—and who can closely acknowledge the patient's contributions, wishes, and circumstances—has to be heavily conditioned by a dose of institutional, professional, and economic reality. Patients' challenges to doctors' calls for compliance (Hasselkus, 1988) and W. Haug and Lavin's (1983) early perceptive remarks on the likelihood of ideologically motivated clashes between consumerism in medical care and help seeking in caregiving, are two such reality doses. The contexts and discourses presented in this special issue also attend to this matter.

Further conditioning factors may be discipline specific, perhaps tied to inherent uncertainties and probabilities in relation to particular conditions and their diagnosis or treatment. For example, the issue of whether professional practitioners provide expert information or expert advice, as in cases of psychotherapy and genetic counseling, or in what circumstances information may count as advice, is not merely a matter of pragmatics; it is centrally connected to participants' identification of expert behavior (C. N. Candlin & Lucas, 1986; Leppanen, 1998; Sarangi, 2000). The expert discursive management of uncertainty, in particular what can and what cannot be announced, is a central theme in this issue in both the article by Sarangi and Clarke and that by Linell et al.

Accordingly, in addressing the issue of how expertise might be realized in discourse, it is appropriate to be cautious. Three factors are in our view important. First, as we indicated earlier and the articles in this special issue evidence, any appraisal of the discourse of expertise needs to be local, site specific, and context specific—even where, as here in relation to the management of risk, the potential exists for cross-site and interdisciplinary analysis. Such location-specific appraisal needs to be further narrowed to particular critical moments within the discipline, activity, and site in question, much as indicated in the articles in this issue. Second, as Linell and his colleagues note in their article, one cannot make the simple assumption that merely because X is held to be an expert, by whatever criteria, therefore what X says is naturally and unproblematically an instance of expert talk. All professional talk is not expert talk, and in many cases, as Sarangi (1998) noted, expertise would appropriately be realized not by talk at all but by strategic silence. Peräkylä warns in his article in this issue, for example, against appraising doctors' expertise simply on the basis of the ways in which they attend to patients' responses. Further, as Sarangi and Roberts (1999a) suggested, distinctions between being expert professionally and being expert institutionally are not necessarily the same thing and may be accompanied by distinctive discourses. In any case, there is no necessary concordance between professional practitioners' own appraisal of expert discourse and that of outside evaluators, be they patients and clients or professional evaluators (Jacoby & McNamara, 1999). Third, we need to be cautious that in identifying discursive features in professional–lay interactions that might be candidates for signaling expert behavior we do not fall into the competency trap of a reductionist identification of expertise to some simple checklist of features. The caution by Cheetham and Chivers (1998) indicated earlier in this introduction is again appropriate here.

Nevertheless, there is compelling evidence from a range of studies in health care and other fields (Buttny, 1996; C. N. Candlin & Garbutt, 1996; C. N. Candlin & Maley, 1994; Drew & Heritage, 1992; Foppa, 1995; Heritage & Sefi, 1992; Maynard, 1991a, 1991b, 1992, 1996; Stivers, 1998) that certain discursive features and discursive strategies do recur in discussions about the relation of discourse to the display of expert behavior. Such features and strategies are best seen as professional resources that accompany or constitute actions, open to be drawn on and linked to particular aspects and displays of professional expertise, and that can be warranted as such by the participants and by other observers. S. Candlin's article in this issue explicitly addresses this matter of members' interactional resources (Fairclough, 1992) in her discussion of nursing expertise. Among these resources is the ability of expert practitioners to manage interactions across distinct planes of discourse—transactional and interactional—and more specifically, their ability to manage complex recontextualizations intertextually and interdiscursively (Adelswärd & Sachs, 1998; C. N. Candlin & Maley, 1997; Linell, 1998; Sarangi, 1998) by employing a variety of voices polyphonically (Bakhtin, 1981) as the context and the expert's shifting roles warrant. Linked to this deployment of recontextualization is a practice that we call *layering* or *staging,* whereby professional expertise relates to the effective control of two discourse trajectories, one strategic and the other tactical. This practice may be especially prevalent in psychotherapeutic discourse (Buttny, 1996; C. N. Candlin & Garbutt, 1996; Davis, 1986) in which the practitioner seeks to move the client gradually toward a point of self-realization of the significance of some event but does so by a sequence of staged tactical actions, each of which falls short of any overt decision or challenge. Davis (1986) wrote of the therapist displaying expertise by highlighting a "problem" quickly and then reformulating this "problem" without disrupting the flow of the interaction. Such a practice appears to be common in other domains, including lawyer–client conferencing (Maley, Candlin, Crichton, & Koster, 1995), family planning counseling (C. N. Candlin & Lucas, 1986), and a clinician breaking bad news to a patient (Maynard, 1991b, 1992). Here professional practitioners gradually prepare for or foreshadow some staged delivery of a diagnosis or conclusion (Maynard, 1992, 1996; Stivers, 1998), or more generally have some ultimate goal for the interaction that they approach by a series of staged steps.

Of all features, perhaps the most prevalent is the reference to the expert's discourse being *recipient designed*. Here the ability referred to is that of tailoring the tenor, content, and management of contributions to match the perceived needs and states of understanding readiness of the patient or client at particular points in the interaction (Drew & Heritage, 1992; Heritage & Sefi, 1992). The effective exercise of such an ability clearly depends on appropriate monitoring by the professional practitioner of the interaction, linked to a flexible adjustment in response to recipient uptake and, as Sarangi and Clarke (2002) indicate, on the appropriately timed reinforcement of mutual knowledge. This matching of response to recipient contribution is characteristic, of course, of many encounters, not only those deemed professional. The issue for the linking of such discursive practice to expertise is in what ways such a practice becomes part of an expert's professional repertoire. Is such "artful reframing" (Buttny, 1996) expert behavior (in the sense we have defined it earlier) or merely the management (however intricate) of good conversational practice?

Recipient design is not merely the prerogative of the professional. In the context of the mandated encouragement of coconstruction by professional practitioners and clients or patients of decisions about courses of action, of the acceptance of diagnoses or analyses, and of agreements about conclusions to be drawn from evidence presented, such discursive features of expertise are jointly rather than unilaterally achieved. The challenge before the expert practitioner as S. Candlin (1997, 2000, 2002) argues is how to develop what she terms *comprehensive coherence*; that is, the gradual making sensible to the professional and the patient or client the nature of their common professionally defined goals. For her, skillful topic management is the key expert resource in the achievement of such coherence.

THE MANAGEMENT OF RISK IN
HEALTH CARE SETTINGS

It has been a theme of this introduction article that definitions of expertise and accounts of the candidate discourses associated with expertise need to be differentiated, particularly in relation to professional sites, local encounters and their themes, and shifting (co)participant roles. At the same time, such definitions and accounts need to be reflected against macrosocial influences both in relation to interprofessional sites and to intraprofessional contexts—for example those pertaining to gender, age, ethnicity, to institutional and professional dysfluencies, and to more socially pervasive conditions, such as the increasing management, technologization, and individualization of late modern society. The theme of risk and the discursive management of risk in health care provides a criterial case for the exploration of these influences and conditioning factors on the display of expertise.

As the articles in this issue indicate, the design and delivery of contemporary health care is profoundly affected by what sociologists and social theorists such as Giddens (1991), Beck (1992), and Luhmann (1993) have referred to as the "risk society," and that anthropologists like Douglas (1990, 1992) see as a society poised between risk and blame. Indeed, Douglas (1992) referred to risk as "becoming a central cultural construct in America" (p. 22) and one that has "entered politics" as it has pervasively entered popular consciousness. Such writers stress the multiple interpretations of risk, seeking to distinguish it, for example, from danger while maintaining a connection to it. Beck (1992) defined risk as a "systematic way of dealing with hazards and insecurities induced and introduced by modernization itself" (p. 21). For Giddens (1991), "the concept of risk becomes fundamental to the ways that lay actors and technical specialists organize the social world" (p. 3). In particular, risk is associated with social and cultural values; "all forms of risk calculation and coping strategy imply a consideration of values and desired ways of life" (Giddens & Pierson, 1998, p. 231). Such linkage of risk with value introduces the key element of the negotiability of risk, in which "a characteristic of the new situations of risk is that the facts of the matter are normally in question and the experts disagree" (Giddens & Pierson, 1998, p. 231). This linkage of risk with negotiation of value is inherently discursive as Adelswärd and Sachs (1998) emphasized when they wrote that it may be not so much the factual basis of risks that are in dispute but rather the interpretations of those facts, and, especially, as a consequence of the manner in which the risks themselves are presented.

It is this assessment of risk as a matter of probabilistic discursive reasoning that has caused some institutions professionally concerned with risk management to seek to constrain and govern the assessment of risk, particularly in contexts of professional judgment and decision making. As one example of such constraints, Firkin and Smith (2002) assessed how risk is evaluated in child protection cases and emphasized the need to see risk assessment as a particular professional and institutional order of discourse, one in which there can be varying degrees of implicit or explicit guidance by agencies as to how experts make judgments and deliver decisions. Here professional expertise in the exercise of judgment over risk is not left to an individual's own expertise but is governed by institutional agency. Expertise has thus become not merely a matter of drawing on professional and lay knowledge and experience (professional status) but also a matter of navigating the frameworks of authority. Firkin and Smith's characterization of risk assessment referring to Boffa and Armitage (1999), as a process of gradual professional decision making calibrated against a range of risk-affecting factors such as severity, vulnerability, likelihood, and safety is well exemplified in the comparative accounts from different "sites of risk" provided by the articles in this issue.

Risk in the context of preventive health care has thus achieved a key, almost iconic status. As Giddens (1991) succinctly put it, "the body is in some sense perennially at risk" (p. 126). He went on to quote Goffman (1972, p. 166) in similar vein stating that "a body is a piece of consequential equipment, and its owner is always putting it on line." Apart from the inherent dubiety about its meanings, risk in the health care context is never unequivocal; its essential polysemy is almost axiomatically associated with difficulties and variability in its expressability. In their study of risk discourse in clinical practice, Adelswärd and Sachs (1998) made the important point (also echoed by Linell et al. in this issue) that professional assessments of risk may be distinct from the ways in which the public at large both talks about and conceptualizes risk. As Lupton (1993) noted, "the rhetoric of risk serves different functions depending on how personally controllable the danger is perceived as being" (p. 430). Risk in doctor–patient interaction, in the life world of the patient, in the world of clinical practice, and in the world of statistics, is not identically formulated. This variability in risk formulation is a thread running through all of the articles in this issue. The close connection between risk and an understanding of the social, and risk as an accompaniment of the delivery of sector-specific health care, is explicitly foregrounded in this issue, providing additional support for linking the micro and the macro, as we have been advocating. In this context, Adelswärd and Sachs (1998) commented that:

> Discursive practices seem to locate risk within, and to make risk a property of the individual instead of constructing risk as one aspect of a hypothetical, complex future event involving numerous interrelated aspects, whereby the event cannot be located precisely—neither in time, space or body. Risk is used rhetorically to present a poten-

tial patient's future as given, in fact as a diagnosis, something that a patient has and suffers from. Risk then becomes what has to be treated. (p. 200)

Their comment resonates precisely with the social analysis of Beck (1992), who wrote:

> [The public] only need to be stuffed full of technical details, and then they will share the expert's viewpoint and assessment of the technical manageability of risks, and thus their lack of risk. Protests, fears, criticism or resistance in the public sphere are a pure problem of information. If the public only knew what the technical people know, they would be put at ease—otherwise they are just hopelessly irrational. (p. 58)

Beck's critical appraisal and his awareness that expertise in the management of risk is not solely—or even primarily—a matter of knowledge but one of discursive negotiation among participant values and experiences, is a leitmotiv of the articles in this special issue. Nor is risk some preexistent given in health care interaction; risk talk can mean both talking about risks and generating risks within talk, and can be initiated by both parties to the interaction. Risk poses a dilemma for professionals (Adelswärd & Sachs, 1998); to talk about risks may exacerbate tensions concerning risk, yet to avoid talk about risk may also lead to anxiety. Risk talk is, accordingly, a risky business for all participants. Primarily, in terms of discourse, this derives from the difficulties surrounding the analysis of the discursive management of uncertainty; the varying entitlements to talk about risk; the conditioning factors of patient condition, treatment, and knowledge; and the timeliness of danger and the likely impact of risk talk.

Two factors, at least, need to be borne in mind continually. First, any such analysis is premised on the identification of contextually specific, and locally drawn on, discourse strategies, which may be differentially available to participants as members' resources (Sarangi, 2000). Second, that display of specialized knowledge, the pronouncement of considered judgments, the response to clients' volunteered information, the maintenance of a nondirective stance in the face of explicit advice seeking, and the reference to other sources of expertise, are all strategies that are themselves inherently matters of risk—in particular, the risk associated with the critical appraisal of cost and benefit. Bourdieu's (1982) *marché linguistique* with its emphasis on the variable and changing rates of exchange of beliefs, attitudes, and knowledge status, has considerable resonance in the study of the discursive management of risk. Calculating those rates of exchange at critical moments in the negotiation of health care is a central issue for the articles that follow.

THIS SPECIAL ISSUE

The first article by Sarangi and Clarke deals with the management of uncertainty in genetics risk communication, focusing on the interlocking relation among expert knowledge systems, the assessment of risk, and the inherent uncertainties associated with genetics counseling. The authors identify the tensions that exist between the genetics counselor and the client in the search for explicit diagnosis, and in so doing highlight the complexity of expert talk. The authors' emphasis on what they refer to as "zones of expertise" importantly localizes the interpretation and evaluation of expertise, and their illustration of how expertise can be displayed by uncertainty indicates how the clinically and therapeutically motivated expression of uncertainty can itself be evidence of expertise. In relation to risk, in their article, they focus on accounting for expert behavior in terms of a resource of discursive strategies drawn on and marshaled at "strategic or critical moments" (C. N. Candlin, 1987) for the display of expertise, suggesting the identification of such moments as an object of professionally directed research inquiry.

S. Candlin's article addresses the evaluation of the behaviors of an expert nurse (who is a registered nurse) compared with those of a less expert assistant in nursing in the context of the assessment of older people in Australia, identifying the achievement of what she terms *comprehensive coherence* as an index of expert performance. Such achievement is premised on an evaluation of the discursive choices made by both participants in the expert practice of achieving therapeutic goals. Risk and uncertainty attend these discursive choices, and S. Candlin is especially concerned with the strategic adjustments to the discourse that both participants need to make to minimize the risk (both to the patient's well-being and the nurse's authority) in making less than adequate assessments. There is, thus, a double jeopardy inherent in the interaction: a risk that the interaction may break down and a risk that an inadequate assessment will be made. The risk for the nurse is located particularly in the distinction that she draws between "social" interaction and "therapeutic" interaction. As with Sarangi and Clarke (2002), S. Candlin also focuses on the strategic resources of both parties, especially identifying topic management and the way that the assessment practices are framed. The selection and deployment of these strategies involve risk that the patient may not disclose essential information (the risk of being misunderstood or of losing face), and therefore, inappropriate or insufficient information will be made available to the professional practitioner.

The article by Linell et al. addresses the key issue of how different contexts of primary health care in Sweden affect expert talk about risk. Their comparison across contexts retains a focus on risk's essentially local identity while offering the potential for making intradisciplinary statements of useful generality. Distinctions between scientific and lay formulations of risk allow them to identify explicit and implicit orientations to risk in talk. Data from their multiple research sites are used to identify a set of risk topics and an array of key factors that affect the way in which risk is talked about in interaction. They show how explanation expresses expertise. In addition, they discuss the compromises that have to be made by professional practitioners among the different demands posed by professional knowledge, by possible personal emotional engagement, and by issues of morality and ethics.

The final article by Peräkylä is concerned with display of expertise by doctors in interactions with patients, and, in particular, with evaluation of the effects of doctors' discursive choices on the quality of patients' responses in primary health care contexts in Finland. Peräkylä finds a strong association between patients' responses and the ways that doctors offer evidence for diagnosis, both in terms of the formulation of such diagnoses and their location within the interaction. Although a regular deference by the patients to doctors' expertise is common to all such patient responses, Peräkylä suggests that different health care systems will be at different points of development (if that is the appropriate term) in the degree of coparticipation and collaboration between professional practitioner and client or patient that they encourage. Such institutional variability will impinge on the nature of discursive interactions and contribute a distinctive flavor to displays of expertise. Of course, this is not only a system-specific matter, as we indicated earlier, but it clearly relates also to specialism, to condition, to site, and to mode of treatment. Peräkylä argues that patients, like doctors, have at their disposal an array of members' strategic resources through which they can offer candidate reasoning from their perspective. To a certain degree, then, patients can display expert behavior, albeit still under the authority of the doctor and within the world defined by the profession of medicine. In his analysis, he shows how patients' extended responses indicate how far and in what ways they can assume specific agency in diagnostic reasoning. For Peräkylä, this exercise of agency counterbalances the doctor's inherent authority as expert. Patients provide an evidential basis for doctors' diagnoses and thereby display a kind of expertise.

The mutual, albeit not equal, display of expertise by professional practitioners and by patients or clients lies at the heart of this special issue. The discourse of risk management is a critical location for the variable display of that mutuality.

REFERENCES

Adelswärd, V., & Sachs, L. (1998). Risk discourse: Recontextualisation of numerical values in clinical practice. *Text, 18,* 191–211.

Bakhtin, M. M. (1981). *The dialogic imagination: Four essays* (M. Holquist, Ed., and C. Emerson & M. Holquist, Trans.). Austin: University of Texas Press.

Beck, U. (1992). *Risk society: Towards a new modernity* (M. Ritter, Trans.). London: Sage.

Benner, P. E. (1984). *From novice to expert: Excellence and power in clinical nursing practice.* Menlo Park, CA: Addison-Wesley.

Boffa, J., & Armitage, E. (1999). *The Victorian risk framework: Developing a professional judgement approach to risk assessment in child protection work.* Unpublished manuscript, Child Protection and Juvenile Justice Branch, Department of Human Services, Melbourne, State of Victoria, Australia.

Bourdieu, P. (1982). *Ce que parler veut dire: L'économie des échanges linguistiques.* Paris: Artheme Fayard.

Buttny, R. (1996). Clients' and therapist's joint construction of the clients' problems. *Research on Language and Social Interaction, 29,* 125–153.

Cameron, R., & Williams, J. (1997). Sentence to ten cents: Case study of relevance and communicative success in non-native–native speaker interactions in a medical setting. *Applied Linguistics, 18,* 415–445.

Candlin, C. N. (1987). Explaining moments of conflict in discourse. In R. Steele & T. Treadgold (Eds.), *Language topics: Essays in honour of Michael Halliday* (pp. 413–429). Amsterdam: Benjamins.

Candlin, C. N. (Ed.). (2002). *Research and practice in professional discourse.* Hong Kong: City University of Hong Kong Press.

Candlin, C. N., & Garbutt, M. (1996, March). *Voicing the self: The role of constructed dialogue in psychotherapy.* Paper presented at the American Association of Applied Linguistics Conference, Baltimore.

Candlin, C. N., & Lucas, J. (1986). Interpretations and explanations in discourse: Modes of "advising" in family planning. In T. Ensink, A. van Essen, & T. van der Geest (Eds.), *Discourse analysis and public life* (pp. 13–38). Dordrecht, The Netherlands: Foris.

Candlin, C. N., & Maley, Y. (1994). Framing the dispute. *International Journal for the Semiotics of Law, 7,* 75–98.

Candlin, C. N., & Maley, Y. (1997). Intertextuality and interdiscursivity in the discourse of alternative dispute resolution. In B.-L. Gunnarsson, P. Linell, & B. Nordberg (Eds.), *The construction of professional discourse* (pp. 201–222). London: Longman.

Candlin, C. N., Moore, A., & Plum, G. (1998, July). *From compliance to concordance: Shifting discourses in HIV medicine.* Paper presented at the Conference of the International Pragmatics Association (IPrA), Rheims, France.

Candlin, S. (1997). *Towards excellence in nursing: An analysis of the discourse of nurses and patients in the context of health assessments.* Unpublished doctoral dissertation, University of Lancaster, Lancaster, England.

Candlin, S. (2000). New dynamics in the nurse–patient relationship? In S. Sarangi & M. Coulthard (Eds.), *Discourse and social life* (pp. 230–245). London: Pearson.

Candlin, S. (2002/this issue). Taking risks: An indicator of expertise? *Research on Language and Social Interaction, 35,* 173–193.

Cheetham, G., & Chivers, G. (1988). The reflective (and competent) practitioner: A model of professional competence which seeks to harmonise the reflective practitioner and competence-based approaches. *Journal of European Industrial Training, 22,* 267–276.

Cicourel, A. (1992). The interpenetration of communicative contexts: Examples from medical encounters. In A. Duranti & C. Goodwin (Eds.), *Rethinking context* (pp. 291–310). Cambridge, England: Cambridge University Press.

Coupland, N., Sarangi, S., & Candlin, C. N. (Eds.). (2001). *Sociolinguistics and social theory.* London: Pearson.

Davis, K. (1986). The process of problem (re)formulation in psychotherapy. *Sociology of Health and Illness, 8,* 44–74.

Deveaux, M. (1994). Feminism and empowerment. *Feminist Studies, 20,* 223–247.

Douglas, M. (1990). Risk as a forensic resource. *Daedalus, 119*(4), 1–16.

Douglas, M. (1992). *Risk and blame: Essays in cultural theory.* London: Routledge.

Drew, P., & Heritage, J. (Eds.). (1992). *Talk at work: Interaction in institutional settings.* Cambridge, England: Cambridge University Press.

Dreyfuss, S. E., & Dreyfuss, H. L. (1980, February). *A five stage model of the mental activities involved in directed skill acquisition.* Unpublished report, Office of Scientific Research, United States Air Force (Contract No. F49620–79–C–0063), University of California, Berkeley.

Fahy, K., & Smith, P. (1999). From the sick role to subject positions: A new approach to the medical encounter. *Health, 3,* 71–93.

Fairclough, N. L. (1992). *Discourse and social change.* Cambridge, England: Polity.

Firkin, A., & Smith, S. (2002). Judgement in child protection practice. In C. N. Candlin (Ed.), *Research and practice in professional discourse.* Hong Kong: City University of Hong Kong Press.

Foppa, K. (1995). On mutual understanding and agreement. In I. Markova, C. Graumann, & K. Foppa (Eds.), *Mutualities in dialogue* (pp. 149–175). Cambridge, England: Cambridge University Press.

Galanti, G. (1991). *Caring for patients from different cultures: Case studies from American hospitals.* Philadelphia: University of Pennsylvania Press.

Giddens, A. (1979). *Central problems in social theory.* London: Macmillan.

Giddens, A. (1990). *The consequences of modernity.* Cambridge, England: Polity.

Giddens, A. (1991). *Modernity and self-identity: Self and society in the late modern age.* Cambridge, England: Polity.

Giddens, A., & Pierson, C. (1998). *Conversations with Anthony Giddens: Making sense of modernity.* Cambridge, England: Polity.

Goffman, E. (1972). *Interaction ritual.* London: Allen Lane.

Hak, T. (1999). "Text" and "con-text": Talk bias in studies of health care work. In S. Sarangi & C. Roberts (Eds.), *Talk, work and institutional order: Discourse in medical, mediation and management settings* (pp. 427–451). Berlin, Germany: Mouton de Gruyter.

Haley, W. E., Clair, J., & Saulsberry, K. (1991). Family caregiver satisfaction with medical care of their demented relatives. *The Gerontologist, 32,* 219–226.

Hasselkus, B. R. (1988). Meaning in family caregiving: Perspectives on caregiver/professional relationships. *The Gerontologist, 28,* 686–691.

Haug, M. R. (1994). Elderly patients, caregivers and physicians: Theory and research on health care triads. *Journal of Health and Social Behavior, 35*(1), 1–12.

Haug, W., & Lavin, B. (1983). *Consumerism in medicine.* Beverly Hills, CA: Sage.

Heritage, J., & Sefi, S. (1992). Dilemmas of advice: Aspects of the delivery and reception of advice in interactions between health visitors and first-time mothers. In P. Drew & J. Heritage (Eds.), *Talk at work: Interaction in institutional settings* (pp. 359–417). Cambridge, England: Cambridge University Press.

Hilbert, R. (1990). Ethnomethodology and the micro–macro order. *American Sociological Review, 55,* 794–808.

Jacoby, S., & McNamara, T. (1999). Locating competence. *English for Specific Purposes, 18,* 213–241.

Kovarsky, D., Duchan, J., & Maxwell, M. (Eds.). (1999). *Constructing (in)competence: Disabling evaluations in clinical and social interaction.* Mahwah, NJ: Lawrence Erlbaum Associates, Inc.

Leppanen, V. (1998). The straightforwardness of advice: Advice-giving in interactions between Swedish district nurses and patients. *Research on Language and Social Interaction, 31,* 209–239.

Linell, P. (1998). Discourse across boundaries: On recontextualisations and the blending of voices in professional discourse. *Text, 18,* 143–157.

Linell, P., Adelswärd, V., Sachs, L., Bredmar, M., & Lindstedt, U. (2002/this issue). Expert talk in medical contexts: Explicit and implicit orientation to risks. *Research on Language and Social Interaction, 35,* 195–218.

Luhmann, N. (1993). *Risk: A sociological theory* (R. Barrett, Trans.). New York: Aldine de Gruyter.

Lupton, D. (1993). Risks as moral danger: The social and political functions of risk discourse in public health. *International Journal of Health Services, 23,* 425–435.

Lynch, M., & Bogen, D. (1994). Harvey Sacks's primitive natural science. *Theory, Culture and Society, 11,* 65–104.

Maley, Y., Candlin, C. N., Crichton, J., & Koster, P. (1995). Orientations in lawyer-client interviews. *Forensic Linguistics, 2,* 42–55.

Maynard, D. (1991a). Interaction and asymmetry in clinical discourse. *American Journal of Sociology, 97,* 448–495.

Maynard, D. (1991b). The perspective-display series and the delivery and receipt of diagnostic news. In D. Boden & D. H. Zimmerman (Eds.), *Talk and social structure* (pp. 164–192). Berkeley: University of California Press.

Maynard, D. (1992). On clinicians co-implicating recipients' perspectives in the delivery of diagnostic news. In P. Drew & J. Heritage (Eds.), *Talk at work: Interaction in institutional settings* (pp. 331–358). Cambridge, England: Cambridge University Press.

Maynard, D. (1996). On "realization" in everyday life: The forecasting of bad news as a social relation. *American Sociological Review, 61,* 109–131.

Mishler, E. G. (1984). *The discourse of medicine: The dialectics of medical interviews.* Norwood, NJ: Ablex.

Moore, A., Candlin, C. N., & Plum, G. (2001). Making sense of viral load: One expert or two? *Culture, Health and Sexuality, 3,* 429–450.

Panagua, F. (1994). *Assessing and treating culturally diverse clients: A practical guide.* Thousand Oaks, CA: Sage.

Parks, J. A. (1998). A contextualised approach to patient autonomy within the therapeutic relationship. *Journal of Medical Humanities, 19,* 299–311.

Peräkylä, A. (2002/this issue). Agency and authority: Extended responses to diagnostic statements in primary care encounters. *Research on Language and Social Interaction, 35,* 219–247.

Royal Pharmaceutical Society of Great Britain. (1997). *From compliance to concordance: Achieving shared goals in medicine-taking.* London: Author.

Sarangi, S. (1998). Rethinking recontextualization in professional discourse studies: An epilogue. *Text, 18,* 301–318.

Sarangi, S. (2000). Activity types, discourse types and interactional hybridity: The case of genetic counselling. In S. Sarangi & M. Coulthard (Eds.), *Discourse and social life* (pp. 1–27). London: Pearson.

Sarangi, S., & Clarke, A. (2002/this issue). Zones of expertise and the management of uncertainty in genetics risk communication. *Research on Language and Social Interaction, 35,* 139–171.

Sarangi, S., & Roberts, C. (1999a). The dynamics of interactional and institutional orders in work-related settings. In S. Sarangi & C. Roberts (Eds.), *Talk, work and institutional order: Discourse in medical, mediation and management settings* (pp. 1–57). Berlin, Germany: Mouton de Gruyter.

Sarangi, S., & Roberts, C. (Eds.). (1999b). *Talk, work and institutional order: Discourse in medical, mediation and management settings.* Berlin, Germany: Mouton de Gruyter.

Schön, D. (1983). *The reflective practitioner: How professionals think in action.* London: Maraca Temple Smith.

Schön, D. (1987). *Educating the reflective practitioner.* San Francisco: Jossey-Bass.

Sherwin, S. (1992). Feminist and medical ethics: Two different approaches to contextual ethics. In H. B. Holmes & L. M. Prude (Eds.), *Feminist perspectives in medical ethics* (pp. 17–31). Indianapolis: Indiana University Press.

Stivers, T. (1998). Pre-diagnostic commentary in veterinarian–client interaction. *Research on Language and Social Interaction, 31,* 241–277.

Warren, M. G., Weitz, R., & Kulis, S. (1998). Physician satisfaction in a changing health care environment: The impact of challenges to professional autonomy, authority and dominance. *Journal of Health & Social Behavior, 39,* 356–367.

Research on Language and Social Interaction, 35(2), 139–171

Zones of Expertise and the Management of Uncertainty in Genetics Risk Communication

Srikant Sarangi
Health Communication Research Centre
Cardiff University

Angus Clarke
University of Wales College of Medicine

In the context of risk communication in genetic counseling, there appears to be a tension between clients seeking an authoritative, definitive risk assessment and the geneticist-expert actively defining the boundaries of his or her (in)expertise through formulation of uncertainty that is such a feature of genetic disorders. In the process of demarcating his or her zone of expertise, he or she defers to the judgment of other medical colleagues with expertise in "adjacent" areas. Our claim is that the genetic counselor delineates his or her (in)expertise through a systematic deployment of a range of modalized discourse strategies (e.g., contrast and hedging) while claiming authority in a limited knowledge field. At the broader professional level, this is motivated in part by the limits to professional knowledge and in part by the desire to maintain a "nondirective" (i.e., neutral) stance. Our analysis focuses on the expert formulation of uncertainty in a single counseling session around 4 strategic moments: (a) display of specialist knowledge, (b) pronouncement of considered judgment, (c) response to clients' volunteered information, and (d) maintenance of a nondirective stance in the face of explicit advice seeking by clients.

Correspondence concerning this article should be sent to Srikant Sarangi, Health Communication Research Centre, Cardiff University, P.O. Box 94, Cardiff CF10 3XB, Wales, UK. E-mail: sarangi@cf.ac.uk

INSTITUTIONAL AND PROFESSIONAL
DIMENSIONS OF EXPERT KNOWLEDGE

One obvious way to look at the general notion of expertise is from the perspective of the phenomenology of knowledge. Schutz (1964) contrasted expert knowledge and lay knowledge as follows:

> The expert's knowledge is restricted to a limited field but therein it is clear and distinct. His opinions are based on warranted assertions: his judgments are not mere guesswork or loose suppositions. The man on the street has a working knowledge of many fields which are not necessarily coherent with one another. His knowledge of recipes indicating how to bring forth in typical situations typical results by typical means. (p. 122)

Expertise, according to this stipulation, implies an in-depth mastery of a field of knowledge. "Warranted assertions" can only be made within a "limited field." Lay knowledge, by contrast, is not distinctly specific: It is rather "typical." Schutz went on to propose that lay perspectives can be mapped onto a continuum—which would be closer to our lived realities. In this view, scientific knowledge, however defined, is no longer a privilege of the experts, and it is becoming increasingly difficult to draw a line between lay and expert knowledge. In the health care domain, Mishler's (1984) dichotomy between the voice of medicine and the voice of the lifeworld may account inadequately now for the progressively less asymmetrical distribution of available knowledge in doctor–patient encounters (Atkinson, 1995; Silverman 1987). Given the rapid advancements in information and technology, the lay public has access to more or less the same kind of scientific knowledge that experts have via surfing of Web sites, participation in support groups, and so on. Indeed the rapid advancement of scientific knowledge makes it difficult for individual professionals to claim expert status in any purist form. The limited field that Schutz referred to suggests the near proximity of or overlapping zones of expertise even within the same profession. In the postmodern society, pluralization of expert knowledge is readily acknowledged and this has consequences for professions such as medicine (Williams & Calnan, 1996).

Moreover, professional knowledge is constituted within a given institutional order (see Sarangi & Roberts, 1999, on the distinction between institutional and professional modes). Whereas the institutional mode is constituted in the abstract, analytic accounts based on scientific knowledge, the professional mode is premised on the practitioner's cumulative experience. Professionals in different institutional contexts strive to retain their control over specialized knowledge, and thus their freedom, by not allowing such knowledge to be routinized (and hence controlled through institutional means). However, what counts as an authoritative professional opinion (i.e., invested with legitimacy) is derived from institutionally sanctioned roles. When one talks about "expert opinion," institutionally sanctioned authority and roles may be a prerequisite to adopting an expert stance. Professional expertise becomes a kind of knowledge and truth claim whereby an expert opinion is regarded as plausible—"more likely to be true than false" (Johnson & Blair, 1983, p. 145). At the interactional level, expert knowledge is manifest in different modes of practice, such as coding, highlighting, and articulating "facts" in professionally specific and institutionally recognizable ways (Goodwin, 1994).

EXPERT RISK ASSESSMENT VIS-À-VIS FORMULATION OF UNCERTAINTY

Our discussion so far suggests that expertise is multifaceted and needs to be narrowly located. When we extend the notion of expertise to the realm of risk assessment, we are immediately faced with issues of uncertainty and probability. The characterization of contemporary Western society as "risk society" (Beck, 1992) is mainly based on the premise that there is typically not sufficient scientific capability (i.e., expertise) to calculate and prevent the eventuation of various risks. In all spheres of life—economy, environment, health—the so-called experts seem to rely increasingly on risk assessment as a prerequisite for action and decision making. Moreover, the expert systems, one could argue, generate risks of all sorts, whether or not they are well-equipped to identify and manage, let alone avoid, presenting risks.

The term *risk*, like *expertise*, is open to multiple interpretations. Douglas (1990, 1992) and Luhmann (1993) offered a useful distinction between risk and danger. For Luhmann, risks are attributable to taking responsibilities and making decisions, whereas danger almost always invokes external attribution. One way of looking at risk is "to take account of the probability of losses and gains" (Douglas, 1990, p. 2). A notion of "avoidable danger" is implied in such a conceptualization. However, according to Bauman (1993), the term *risk* "belongs to the discourse of gambling, that is, to a kind of discourse which does not sustain clear-cut opposition between success and failure, safety and danger" (p. 200). This suggests that uncertainty is an integral component of risk, and so a cost–benefit analysis of losses and gains as the basis for deciding on action may not be sufficient. As Douglas (1986) rightly pointed out, "a great deal of risk analysis is concerned with trying to turn uncertainties into probabilities" (p. 42). According to Hacking (1975), assessment of risk relies heavily on probabilistic reasoning of two kinds: (a) an appraisal of degrees of belief and evidence; and (b) the tendency of populations to produce "stable, relative frequencies" of events. The first kind relates to what we take as expressions of uncertainty, whereas the latter refers to how individual risks are compared against standard levels. In the context of genetic counseling, as we will see later, these two dimensions of probability are discursively realized through the use of epistemic modalities and appeals to population risk figures.

Uncertainty is integral to the domain of health and illness—both for lay patients and for expert professionals. As Hughes (1958/1981) put it:

> The layman has to learn to live with the uncertainty if not of ignorance, at least of lack of technical knowledge of his own illnesses; the physician has to live with and act in spite of the more closely calculated uncertainty that comes with knowing the limits of medical knowledge and his own skill. (p. 120)

This aligns with Atkinson's (1995) characterization of expertise in terms of how "precisely the physician *locates* the sources and nature of doubt, equivocation and the like" (p. 122):

> It is undoubtedly the case that medical students and practitioners make frequent appeals to matters of opinion, or judgment that cannot be validated unambiguously by scientific knowledge. But personal knowledge and experience are not normally treated by practitioners as reflections of uncertainty, but as warrants for certainty. (Atkinson, 1995, p. 114)

For medical professionals, then, it becomes not a matter of managing uncertainty, but rather a matter of conveying the grounds for the uncertainty—and this entails the demonstration of what is known (i.e., certain).

According to Fox (1957), there are two basic types of uncertainty: (a) incomplete or imperfect mastery of available knowledge and (b) limitations in current medical knowledge. Fox went on to argue that a third source of uncertainty derives from the preceding two: "This consists of difficulty in distinguishing between personal ignorance or ineptitude and the limitations of present medical knowledge" (pp. 208–209). It is likely that mature physicians would attribute uncertainty to limitations in current medical knowledge, whereas a student doctor is more likely to put it down to (a). Also, the level of uncertainty varies according to different subspecialities within medicine (Atkinson, 1999). We would suggest that in the case of genetics, (b) is very much the case, but of course (b) directly impacts on (a) when we take into account everyday counseling practice.

THE POSITIONING OF THE EXPERT IN GENETICS RISK COMMUNICATION

The interlocking relation between expert knowledge systems, risk assessment, and uncertainty provides an apt backdrop for our discussion of genetic counseling. In recent years, counseling—both as a discourse type and as a discursive site—has attracted enormous attention from discourse and communication scholars (e.g., Candlin & Lucas, 1986; Greatbatch & Dingwall, 1999; Jefferson & Lee, 1981; Labov & Fanshel, 1977; Peräkylä, 1995; Silverman, 1997). The professional status of counselors may vary from one setting to another, as would be the kinds of "troubles telling" that clients bring to such encounters. It is inevitable, therefore, that counseling professionals will draw selectively on a body of specialist knowledge within a given institutional order, supplementing such knowledge with episodes of personal or professional opinion.

Genetic counseling is a complex speech activity in which professionals and clients discuss issues related to disorders that are, or may be, genetic in origin. Referrals for clinical genetic assessment are made by other professionals for three principal reasons, any or all of which may be topics discussed in genetic counseling clinics. These common reasons for referral are (a) the wish to have firm diagnostic or prognostic information about a problem affecting one or more individuals in the family, especially a diagnostic label; (b) the wish for information about the chance of a genetic disorder developing in a so far unaffected member of the family, perhaps the person referred; or (c) the desire for information about the chance of a future child being affected by a congenital or childhood-onset condition.

Discussions that begin with these topics often wander onto different terrain and address a range of related topics, such as the way in which the family disorder came to attention, the possibilities for predictive genetic testing or prenatal diagnosis, surveillance to detect early signs of a disorder or to avoid its complications, a couple's desire to have (further) children, the type of support that can be provided for affected individuals, or the responses of other family members to their genetic situation.

These clinic discussions therefore contain many different elements and remain a hybrid speech event (Sarangi, 2000a). The professional gathers relevant information, including the nature of the client's concerns and the ways in which family members have been affected. Clients may wish to find out more in general terms about their particular condition or they may have specific issues to address. For example, if a client is confronting a decision about prenatal or predictive testing, then the conversation is likely to address how he or she would respond to the various possible scenarios that may lie ahead—such as having a favorable test result, or an unfavorable result, or deciding not to proceed with testing. Genetic counseling could therefore be expected to consist largely of family background and personal context provided by the client and of technical information provided by the counselor—but it is not so simple.[1]

Uncertainty is a major, but neglected, topic in genetic counseling (van Zuuren, van Essen, & van der Geest, 1997; see also Clarke, 1991, 1997; Michie, Bron, Bobrow, & Marteau, 1997). There may be uncertainty about the diagnosis of the condition causing concern in the family; many children with developmental problems never have a satisfactory diagnosis provided despite full medical assessment. It is not merely that the particular professional cannot make the diagnosis but that there is no diagnosis to be made (see our preceding discussion of Fox, 1957). Accordingly, the professional may appeal to various sources of evidence to justify this state of affairs—to colleagues, to lay organizations, to the medical literature, and so forth. The professional may share some of his or her (in)expertise to account for the inevitable uncertainty and this may heighten the lack of credibility of his or her expert role.

The information that is provided in a genetic counseling clinic, whether or not a diagnosis has been established, is often risk information—and hence necessarily an expression of uncertainty surrounding future events. Talk about the progress of a disease, whether a future child will or will not be affected by a feared disease, whether the client will or will not develop a degenerative illness or a cancer amounts to focusing on the risk and probability of such events. Even when apparent certainty is available—"I am afraid to say that you do carry the Huntington's disease mutation"—there will still be uncertainty about when and how the mutation may begin to cause frank disease or how the illness will progress in someone who has begun to show signs of the disorder. The questions that really concern a family, therefore, may not be answerable with certainty—even when there are plenty of hard, objective medical facts known about the condition. This is especially the case in the evaluation of reproductive risks (Parsons & Atkinson, 1992, 1993). The numerical risk value (probability) of the adverse future event may not be of much interest to the client, who may only be interested in the dichotomous outcome (either it will or it will not happen), but a focus on probability does give the professional scope for precision, or at least the appearance of precision (Sarangi, 2002). Attention to risk can then be seen as a professional strategy for retaining the authority of an expert in the face of uncertainty. What emerges is a complex scenario regarding expert talk about uncertainty while assessing and communicating risk.

FORMULATION OF GENETIC EXPERTISE
THROUGH DISCOURSE STRATEGIES

In this article, we offer a detailed analysis of a single clinical genetic encounter to show how the expert geneticist manages the various dimensions of uncertainty as discussed previously. Our main concern was to examine the discourse strategies that experts (in this case, genetic counselors) and their clients use to deal with the notion of risk assessment. We argue that a range of discursive resources are mobilized—ranging from explicit formulations of claiming insufficient knowledge (e.g., "I don't know"), reference to other sources of expertise (e.g., "X is better placed to comment on this"), and use of hedges (e.g., "I'm not sure but . . .") to deployment of rhetorical strategies such as contrast (Sarangi & Clarke, 2002) and reinforcement of mutual knowledge (see Sarangi, 2000b, on the strategic use of A/B events). Our analysis here focuses on how (dis)claiming of knowledge is accomplished through the delineation of different zones of expertise and the accompanying use of contrast and hedging devices. First, there is the need for a demarcation of the specialist's territory and its distinction from the territories of other medical specialists.[2] This is what Hughes (1958/1981) referred to as "there being subcultures within the greater professional medical cultures": "This is also more than a matter of technique and knowledge; it has roots in ideas and assumptions" (p. 118). The expert (here the geneticist) has to disclaim ownership of scientific knowledge of certain kind and, when necessary, defer risk assessment to other specialists. This is a form of role distancing. Expressions such as "I am not a neurosurgeon" can act as a marker of where the geneticist's zone of expertise ends and that of the neurosurgeon begins.

On the whole, interactional demarcation of zone of expertise has to do with assessments of what has been just said or is about to be said (Pomerantz, 1984). If the geneticist prefaces his or her assessment of the situation with "I am not a neurosurgeon," what she or he says next needs to be interpreted within this frame of professed inexpertise. Although assessments are a feature of everyday talk, they assume specific significance in the institutional setting, mainly because of the potential uptake of the information and explanation that counselors provide. It is quite possible that hedged expressions such as "you might want to think about doing X," despite the preceding disclaimer "I am not a neurosurgeon," could be heard by patients as explicit advice because of the authority and position of speaking generally associated with medical professionals. This requires an examination of the complex relationship between giving information and giving advice, because advice can be packaged as information and vice versa (Candlin & Lucas, 1986; Sarangi, 2000a; Silverman, 1997).

The formulation of uncertainty through hedging can be identified at a local level. Numerical formulations of risk provide an opportunity to display precision, but in many settings—wherever there is uncertainty about the probabilities—they are accompanied by indications of hedging and may be followed by illustrations and disclaimers. Hedging can then be seen as a framing device to introduce evidence (perhaps based on recent research findings) and as a way of taking an expert position to evaluate such (numerical) evidence in the context of the case in hand (see Hacking, 1975, previously). Risk information may be disclaimed in the same turn as being asserted (e.g., I may be wrong but the risk is fifty–fifty). The claim (risk is fifty–fifty) is thus qualified. Evaluative discourse and information go hand in hand.[3] As Hopper and colleagues (Hopper, Ward, Thomason, & Sias, 1995) pointed out in the context of Cancer Information Service, nonmedical health information officials are institutionally required to use disclaimers. These are situations in which information can be provided but not advice. In other words, the information falls short of a claim because of the use of disclaimers (whether as early disclaimers or embedded disclaimers[4]).

The occurrence of hedging in professionals' talk is intricately linked to the discourse of (im)precision, and by extension, to that of uncertainty. In an extensive study of biomedical slide talks, Dubois (1987) offered a taxonomy of various modalities deployed by scientists to formulate imprecision. These include verbs (e.g., *think, suggest, guess*), auxiliaries (e.g., *might, may, could*), nouns (e.g., *estimate*), adverbs (e.g., *roughly, approximately, about*), and so forth. Other discourse features under imprecision include, for example, extreme rounding, ranges, and so forth. The title of Dubois's article, "Something on the Order of Around Forty to Forty Four" is a good illustration of "imprecision raised to the fourth power." In other linguistics–pragmatics research, two types of hedging disclaimers have been identified (Prince, Frader, & Bosk, 1982): approximator ("sort of," "nearly") and the shield ("I'm not sure," "as far as I know"). The shield can be of two kinds: plausibility shield (uncertain reasoning) and attribution shield (citing a source). Wachtel (1980) provided a comprehensive account of approximators in terms of their pragmatic functions versus semantic differences. Many of these taxonomic accounts of hedging and approximators are not interactionally grounded, but as we see in our analysis, these devices are selectively drawn on by both professionals and clients in the counseling context. Relevant here is the observation made by Beach and Metzger (1997) about how people claim insufficient knowledge through formulation of "I don't know"—both in everyday and institutional contexts—(a) to mark uncertainty about next-positioned response; (b) to construct neutral positions by mitigating agreement or disagreement, disattending, and seeking closure to other-initiated topics; and (c) to postpone or withhold acceptance of others' invited or requested actions.

In identifying this linkage between delineation of expertise (mainly through contrast) and the formulation of uncertainty (mainly through hedging), our aim here is to examine their interactional manifestation in the context of the counseling activity. In the final part, we provide some reasons as to what other factors (besides the lack of current knowledge) might be the source of formulations of uncertainty. We suggest that geneticists' commitment to nondirectiveness may be a crucial factor. The genetic counselor may be reluctant to dispense overt advice because this would breach the professional code of nondirectiveness. Uncertainty and nondirectiveness go hand in hand, and therefore professional action in terms of advice giving is not always possible in genetic counseling clinics. By focusing on a single case we hope to be able to capture the cumulative way in which formulations of uncertainty and zones of (in)expertise unfold during interaction. The clinic consists of the geneticist (D) and a couple (W = wife, H = husband). W, who is in her mid-30s, had a meningioma removed 2 years previously and she is concerned about its recurrence in future pregnancy. This is their first visit to the genetics clinic, and they have not been visited by a specialist nurse at home to discuss preliminaries (such preclinic contact is the preferred practice in this clinic).

DATA ANALYSIS

At the opening stages (originally lines 33–56) W and H take turns to summarize the present medical condition,[5] and in doing so they allude to the notion of delineation of different zones of medical expertise (see Appendix for an overall tracking of the initiation and scope of (in)expertise as formulated by the three participants):

Example 1

01   W: [. . .] we went to the eh eh consultant for a routine interview
02   D: yeah
03   W: after an MRI
04   D: yeah
05   W: yeah (.) and eh we spoke about pregnancy and (.) he thinks
          it's not a good idea to get pregnant now straightaway (.) I
          should wait for two years (.) well I- am I turn thirty five and I'm
          I'm a bit worried you know regarding age (.) you know with
          all the things you hear about (.) you know the longer you leave
          it the more this and that (.) so eh (.) he said well it I'm not
          the best person to ask your- to answer your question he said
          see you should see the genetic people (.5) so eh you know (.)
          although the the mister (doctor's name) the one who
          performed the actual operation he felt there is no harm in
          getting pregnant or trying to get pregnant (.) you know and eh
          (.) don't know why he came up with this opinion (.) but

anyway (.) I spoke to my GP (.) in our local surgery and he
said eh (.) he sent us here (.) He doesn't think there is eh
anything eh <u>dangerous</u> to go ahead with the idea of pregnancy
but eh (.5) he thought he might take his eh (.) you know
opinion into consideration so he referred me (.) but <u>he</u>
<u>personally doesn't think</u> there is anything eh (.) you know
⌐(.) any danger ⌐
06   H: ⌐we actually had⌐ conflicting eh eh feedback when we
asked people about eh the danger of a recurrence of the
meningioma

07   D: yes

08   H: being being it it feeds of the eh::: (.) eh the hormonic changes
in a woman's body when she's pregnant (.) and they said
there's there <u>is</u> a chance that it could come back (.5) eh you
know suppose it doesn't can't come back in one go because it's
a slow growing tumor but (it gives it a good) (.5) kickstart (.) if
there's anything left

Here W and H juxtapose the various expert opinions in relation to the
risks associated with W's second pregnancy. The uncertainties are manifest
through these differing opinions and it is hoped that a genetic perspective
might help to resolve the situation. The consultant (senior neurosurgeon),
the more junior neurosurgeon (who performed the surgery), and the general
practitioner (GP) have already offered their own evaluations of W's
current condition and the implications this may have for future pregnancies. In fact, both the junior neurosurgeon and the GP share the view that
an immediate pregnancy does not have any associated risk. The consultant, by contrast, thinks otherwise: "It's not a good idea to get pregnant
now straightaway" (turn 5). Notice that W recruits the various expert opinions through different discoursal means. The opinion of the consultant is
expressed through direct speech (e.g., "I'm not the best person to answer
your . . . question," "you should see the genetic people . . ."). This direct
quote serves to authorize why they are seeking the expert views of a geneticist. Notice how, in turn 5, the GP's opinion is repeated in an emphatic
way, although the second formulation is qualified with "<u>he personally</u>
<u>doesn't think</u>." Both W and H, however, display a competent understand-
ing of their medical condition, as they seek a precise formulation of the
risks associated with a future pregnancy.

A little later (originally lines 174–188) D gives his opinion:

Example 2

01 D: yeah. 'cause I don't- I don't think there's any reason to think
        that (.) a pregnancy could (.) eh (.) make the difference
        between a recurrence or not a recurrence (.5) I think (.) it
        might not- I suppose it <u>might</u> influence the rate of growth of a
        proper (.) eh tumor (.) so that if there was a small recurrence
        then it might show itself a little bit sooner. (.) but that's only a
        a might (.) and eh (.) .hhh I think really from the point of
        view of the tumor you had (.) I think the normal MRI scan
        you've had since this (.) offers you a lot of reassurance (0.7)
        eh (.) and (.) I don't I don't think I am really I'm in- (0.7) I
        am in I'm not in a good position to (.) to <u>advise</u> and the I think
        Mr (name)- (.) the neurosurgeons (.) you know (.) are going to
        have a much better (.)

02 W: mmh

03 D: idea as to how <u>likely</u> it is to come back (.) and if Mr. (name) is
        fairly confident (.) that he managed to remove it all, and if the
        MRI scan has been normal then hhhh (0.5)

04 W: I don't know <u>why</u> he said that he maybe (.) ehm you know it's
        all confused

At the surface level, D here recruits a range of hedging devices (*I think, I suppose, might, from the point of view, likely, a little bit sooner,* etc.). The long pauses are also an indication of uncertain reasoning, but note the expression "that's only a might," which is a rather forceful assertion under the circumstances. Nonetheless, D explicitly defers to the neurosurgeon, who is better placed to ascertain the successful removal of the earlier tumor. He highlights the MRI scan as the basis for reassurance, however. It is on the basis of this evidence that an accurate prediction about (non)recurrence can be made. By default, D discredits the consultant neurosurgeon's concerns, but this is not explicitly commented on. There is, however, the explicit formulation of his nonexpert status ("I'm not in a good position to . . . <u>advise</u>"). Notice, however, that although it is both the GP and the junior neurosurgeon who have voiced a positive opinion about the immediate pregnancy (similar to what the geneticist says here), D recruits the more authoritative voice of the neurosurgical colleagues, rather than that of the GP, to endorse his own opinion. It is a strategic combination of nondirectiveness and an appeal to division of expert labor.

A little later (originally lines 249–266), D further emphasizes his zones of expertise vis-à-vis that of the neurosurgeon.

Example 3

01 D: =yeah you can use steroids to (.) reduce the swelling (.) but-
(.) but (.) but this sort of question I can give some answers to
(.) but (.) eh:::: (.) but (.) it's not (.) my (.) it's just not my
field really (.) and I think that the neurosurgeons who (.)
diagnosed it and treated it

02 W: mmh

03 D: are are the right people to be telling you about .hhhh (.5) eh
(1.5) how how another (.) tumor might show itself (.) if you
had a recurrence (.) they're the right people to be saying how
it might show (.) and what the best treatment would be if that
did happen

04 W: mmh

05 D: (.) I- I see no reason why (.) the question of- why pregnancy
(.) I don't see how that could make any difference to whether
or not a recurrence happens (.) I can see it might make a
slight difference to (.) how quickly it will show, (.) and so- if if
eh - quite a lot of tumors (.) the rate of growth will (.) vary
with (.) ehm hormonal- factors

06 W: mmh

07 D: and (.) so (.5) ehm I think I've heard that meningiomas
sometimes will be influenced a little bit by pregnancy (.) but-
.hhhhh (.) eh so I can imagine that having a pregnancy might
(.) bring the signs of the tumor recurring forward a little bit,
but I don't think it would make- I wouldn't expect it to make a
big difference (.) but that's something where the opinions of
the neurosurgeons really

08 W: mmh

09 D: would be- would make much more sense

What emerges from the preceding are the statements about insufficient knowledge and that somebody knows better. This is different from Beach and Metzger's (1997) interactional account. In health care contexts, the "I don't know" positions have to be qualified by saying who else knows better and by giving some qualified assessments of clients' questions rather than just a shift of topic. Unlike everyday assessments, here we have clients who—rightly or wrongly—assume that the experts know best.

In what follows we select an extended sequence (Examples 4–7) from the later part of the clinic (following the discussion of family tree, originally lines 325–545) to focus on how the geneticist expert discoursally accomplishes the delineation of his zones of expertise vis-à-vis the uncertainty associated with this particular case. Our choice is motivated by the following criteria as far as display of professional expertise is concerned:

1. A first critical moment (Example 4) that represents a genuine information-giving sequence such as what genes are and what causes certain conditions. This counts toward an authoritative display of specialist genetic knowledge, which the clients may or may not have access to before they come to the clinic.

2. A second critical moment (Example 5) in which the geneticist meticulously studies the available facts and goes on to pronounce a considered judgment. This is similar to the mainstream diagnostic phase of medical consultation. In our case, this involves looking at the family tree and making an evaluation of the risk of inheritance of the tumor.

3. A third critical moment (Example 6) is when patients and clients volunteer additional information about their situation, rather unexpectedly, but expect the professional to deal with such information. In these contexts, professional expertise has to be managed in a contingent manner. In our data, this happens when H wants to find out if W's accidental fall when she was a child will have anything to do with recurrence of tumor.

4. A final critical moment (Example 7) is when the clients implicitly or explicitly seek advice about a future course of action. The challenge for the professional counselor is to deal with this request in a nondirective way, but without undermining his or her expert status.

In the following excerpt, D underlines his expertise by suggesting how skin patches can be linked to a particular form of meningioma. This then provides the basis for a physical examination of W[6] and a discussion about family members to ascertain if this genetic condition runs in the family. The discourse thus assumes the status of a genetics perspective as the focus shifts from recurrence of the tumor during pregnancy to its inheritance in the family.

Example 4: Display of specialist knowledge

01 D: so in the absence of (.) anyone else seeming to have eh (.)
        tumors like this (.) then then that (.) eh (.) the chance of there
        being any sort of predisposition to it is small (.) there is-
        there's probably one (.) specific eh (.) condition that is
        probably (.) probably just about worth looking (.) eh (.) which
        is very unlikely but I imagine is what the neurosurgeon was
        thinking about when he said- when he suggested that you saw
        someone in genetics (.) .hhhh eh - and (.) that's a condition
        that sometimes will cause (.) eh (.5) little patches on the skin

02 W: mmh=

03 D: =eh (.) eh (.) slightly darker skin patches (.) and (.)
        sometimes cause eh (.) something in the (.) lens of the eye
        that is not a problem {H: yeah} but can be looked for (.) as a-
        as a sign if you like for the condition and (.5) .hhhhh (.) so we
        have- do you know if you have any- (.) I mean everyone has a
        few little skin marks=

04 W: =mmh=

05 D: =but do you- do you have particular skin marks
        (.5)

06 D: no (.) no

07 W: no

08 D: okay (.5) .hhhh eh (.) now it depends how - how thorough I
        want to be about this (.) I could- do you have no freckles or
        anything (.) no little marks on the skin

09 H: are these (tell-the tale) signs of a (.) for a recurrence or or-
        (1.0)

10 D: hmm not for a recurrence (.) but there is- there is a particular
        but un- very unusual condition that eh (.) can cause
        meningiomas (.) and also give little marks on the skin

11 W: mmh=

12 D: =but (.) I think if you don't have-

13 W: ehm ehm

14 H: (what about) that little little growth on your neck ⌐(unclear)

15 W: └n::yeah a
        mole you know
        ((D goes over to have a look at W's neck))

16 H: tiny little ones growing back to one side=

17   D: =yes (.) that's nothing. (.) yeah that's nothing that's just [very
          (.) very average

At the surface level, this is very much a dispensing of expert knowledge—both at factual and probabilistic levels. In some instances, the information is textbook knowledge, but it can be used strategically (as we
will see in Example 6) to dispel unnecessary anxiety. In turn 1, D uses the
evidence from family history to formulate his zone of expertise. Instead of
talking about recurrence of the tumor during pregnancy, he now talks
about "predisposition" in the family—and this evaluation aligns with his
expertise. Not only does he recontextualize the clients' concerns (from recurrence of the tumor during pregnancy to predispositions to tumors like
this in the family), he is also able to reformulate the neurosurgeon's concern into a possible genetic condition based on skin marks. This is then an
expert reading of a coprofessional's reasoning for a referral. The elicitation sequence in turns 3, 5, and 8 is thus legitimated. In turn 9, H makes an
attempt to return to the theme of recurrence of the tumor, but this is in-
stantly foiled by D as he tries to clarify that what he is talking about is the
link between very unusual skin marks and a form of meningioma. The geneticist's zone of expertise also extends to making distinctions between
little moles and different kinds of skin marks (see turns 3–5 and turn 17).
     The next excerpt follows from the previous example (with a few turns
omitted).

Example 5: Putting the pieces together

01   D: but given that there's nothing (.) nothing in the family (.) and
          that there are no- no signs of this unusual (.) very rare
          condition that will sometimes cause (.) meningiomas
02   W: hm mhm
03   D: and can run in the family (.) I mean given that then (.) from-
          from my point of view I mean there's no (.5) eh::::: (.5) there's
          no reason to think (.) that this is anything but a (.) one-off ⌐(.)
          event
04   W: └mmh mmh
05   D: =that's (.) happened (.) out of the blue and (.) eh (1.5) I can't
          comment on the risk of recurrence (.) because that has to do
          with the neurosurgery and (.) did they take it all out - or not.
          (.5) but I- I can say that the chance of (.) a separate tumor

```
                    happening again (.) not a recurrence but a different one (.) or
                    (.) a- a- tumor in other members of the family is sm- is tiny
06    W:    mhm
07    D:    you know and it isn't really- (.) it's not increased (.) I mean
                    anyone has a chance of a tumor
08    W:    mmh
09    D:    of some sort but there's no reason to think that (.) this
                    happening in you would increase the risk (.) of tumors in other
                    people in the family (.) or in yourself
                    (1.5)
10    D:    ┌such as-
11    W:    └just bad luck (slight laugh)
                    (.)
12    D:    ye::::::s. (.5) yes effectively.
                    (1.0)
13    H:    does eh- does (W's name) have more of a chance (.) of it (.)
                    occurring a- brand new in another area? (.) because she had
                    one or is is- (.) we're back to square one, it's ┌just like anybody
                    else                                                                                     │
14    D:                                                                    └yeah =you- you're
                    virtually back to square one.
15    H:    mhm
16    D:    I mean I think (.) ehm (.5) there's no (.) eh (.5)
17    W:    guarantee=
18    D:    =well I suppose (.) hhhh (.) with it having happened once (.) I
                    suppose there's a a sl- a slight chance that it's (.) eh (.5) that
                    the chance - there must be a small chance
19    W:    mhm hm
20    D:    of it (.) of there having been some reason for that that hasn't
                    been identified. (.) and that (.) so it's not- (.) ca- I can't say that
                    the chance of another one coming is (.) absolutely back to the
                    chance of (.5) uhm that other people have in the population. (.)
                    I can't I can't say it's quite that small.=
21    W:    =mmh mmh=
22    D:    =but it is very small (2.0)
```

In turn 1, we see D interpreting the information about family tree[7] but formulating it as "from my point of view"—which is the genetics point of view. Such a formulation functions as a "shield" (Prince et al., 1982). It is a hedged response to the facts available for interpretation (a potential contrast is suggested between this point of view and that of the neurosurgeon in turn 5). The "warranted assertion" is based on the fact that there is nothing on the family side (see turns 1 and 3; the linguistic formulation "given that" as evidential marking, with further mitigation such as "I mean" and "from my point of view"). Here is a contrast between past and future running in the family, and the issue of recurrence is contrasted with the tumor being a "one-off event, . . . happened out of the blue." We can also see the two dimensions of probabilistic reasoning that Hacking (1975) talked about. Expressions such as "there's no reason to think" (turn 9) and "there having been some reason for that" (turn 20) reiterate the evidential stance introduced early on in turn 1 ("given that"). In turn 20, D also alludes to the standard population trends to reassess the individual risk as "[not] quite that small . . . but it is very small" (turns 20–22).

D suggests, in turn 5, that the neurosurgeon is better placed to comment on risk of recurrence, thereby implying that he can talk only about risks associated with inheritance. This form of disclaimer, accomplished via role distancing, helps to establish the fact that the genetics point of view is one among many possible interpretations. Whereas the issue of inheritance relates to family history, the issue of recurrence relates to the history of the tumor itself ("did they take it all out?"). If the tumor, rather than the patient and the family tree, is the focus of expert scrutiny, then a different knowledge base—that of the neurosurgeon—has to be appealed to for predicting future events. In this turn we also see a further contrast between a separate tumor appearing in the brain versus the recurrence of the same tumor. Everyday normality is appealed to in the formulation "anyone has a chance of a tumor . . . of some sort" (turns 7–9). From a genetics perspective, therefore, it would make sense to talk specifically about recurrence versus inheritance.

The contrast is thus narrowed down to one between (a) the original tumor recurring, (b) a new tumor developing in the mother's case, or (c) the unborn child inheriting one (which is one of the concerns here with regard to pregnancy: whether pregnancy would trigger any of these processes). This kind of discriminatory assessment of facts and evidence through contrastive formulations not only aims for clarity of exposition; it is also constitutive of professional expertise and knowledge. D is more likely to comment on the basis of what the family tree shows and by assuming that the surgery was fully satisfactory. Therefore, his comments are more to do with the risks posed for the unborn child (turn 9) than about recurrence of tumor in mother—the latter clearly falls within the remit of the neurosurgeon.

We then move into a contrastive assessment of chance versus recurrence. In turn 13, H poses a question that is information seeking (e.g., "a-brand new in another area . . . we're back to square one, it's just like anybody else"). D concurs with this by giving an answer, formulated as information with some certainty ("you're <u>virtually</u> back to square one"). The uncertainty, however, is realized through pauses and halted speech (turn 16). W's completion of D's previous turn with "guarantee" in turn 17 is somewhat indicative of D's uncertainty and reluctance to be categorical, as well as W's willingness to go along with D's assessment of the situation. In turns 18–20, D revises his earlier assessment of uncertainty—with a noticeable shift from risk to chance. He now puts W as a bit different from others, again as part of professional discrimination (turn 9), using a contrast between specific case and population—which is a typical contrast pattern in genetic counseling.

Our next example marks a critical juncture in which, out of uncertainty, the clients volunteer additional information either to see if such "new" information would help in the risk assessment or simply to put their minds at ease if such information turned out to be irrelevant. In a sense, one could view Example 5 as a potential closure, with the geneticist having exhausted all possible explanations. At such a moment, volunteering of additional information by clients stretches the encounter to bring off another attempt at resolving uncertainty, as it again calls for an incremental assessment of the situation by the counselor. The following extract continues from Example 5.

Example 6: Formulating an alternative

23 H: I've heard one of the causes well (.) <u>possible</u> causes was (.) an
         impact to the head (.5) and that eh people who'd had head
         injuries they (.) there was a re- research some years ago (.)
         and they found out that where the skull had cracked (.) on the
         inside of the skull (.)=

24 D: =right=

25 H: =ehm in many cases they had a a a growth (.)

26 D: a meningioma?=

27 H: =a meningioma then it was discarded because they said there
         wasn't enough information (.) I don't know if you heard of it
         (.) 'cause (W's name) remembers (.) having a horrendous (.)
         hit on the back of her head (.) when she was a child on the
         same spot where (.5) where she had the tumor

28 W: We were playing and ⌐running after each other ⌐but I came
        against a ⌐rope ⌐and=   [
29 H: [⌐ so we were wondering- ⌐
                          ⌐yeah⌐

30 W: =I didn't see it (.) and it hit me here and I went back on the
        concrete ⌐but
31 H: ⌐how much quick (unclear)
32 W: I didn't faint or anything] at the time (.) but I remember falling
        because it was so eh (.) but that's when I was ten years old
33 D: right (.) I- (.) .hhhh eh:::: hhhhhhhh (.) I=
34 W: =I don't know
35 D: I'd- (.) I'd be quite interested to know what the neurosurgeons
        think (.) I think- I don't think ⌐I know-
36 H: ⌐actually I asked
        him
37 D: what did he say?
38 H: he told me that research (.) he heard of- he heard of it
        because I read it in a book in Blackwells (.) and eh (.) he said
        eh that ⌐research was discarded.
39 D: ⌐right
40 H: 'cause there wasn't enough evidence
        (.5)
41 D: right I mean you can (.) sort of imagine if there's some injury
        (.5) eh (.5) something that makes the the meninges (.) you
        know the- these membranes
42 H: mhm hm
43 D: have to grow (.5) so if- like an injury being a stimulus to them
        to- to heal and grow if there's been some- some damage but
        (.) eh (.) the chance of that (.5) whether there'd be enough
        damage to cause that without it really eh (.5) how can I put it
        (.) .hhhh causing you more than a sore head
44 W: mmh mmh
45 D: eh (.) that sounds a bit unlikely but I
46 H: mmh
47 D: would imagine at least if there's a fracture there or something
48 W: mmh hm
49 D: it's a bit easier to imagine that you've got tissue having to- (.)
        cells having to divide and grow a bit
50 H: mhm

51   D: to heal over

52   H: mmh

53   D: and maybe that (.) that simulation of growth carries on longer
          than it should and becomes a tumor (unclear)=

54   H: =that was the-=

55   D: =yeah (.) but- but if if this injury you had (.) didn't (.) if it
          didn't cause a fracture and didn't cause (.) (unclear) quite
          serious problems at the time then it's a bit harder to know but
          I .hhhh

In turn 23, H volunteers information based on a research article, but he is quick to dismiss the findings because of lack of supportive evidence. Here we see an illustration of clients having access to expert knowledge (a display of information + assessment). H initiates a narrative about W's fall when she was 10 years old and had a hit on her head, on the same spot where she had the tumor. W continues the narrative, filling it with all the exact details about how the accident happened. It is H who keeps interrupting W's narrative (turns 28–32) to signal his motivation behind bringing up this new information—whether there is a link to be established between this fall and the risk of recurrence of the tumor (cf. turn 29: "so we were wondering"). Here they are both talking about the tumor that has been operated on. If a link can be established between the accident and the tumor, it could mean a reduction in uncertainty about the recurrence versus inheritance (see Example 5 previously).

As far as W and H are concerned, there is the expectation that D would now be able to offer a more considered, expert assessment. We notice, in turn 33, D showing hesitation. W's "I don't know" in turn 34 signals an appeal for some confirmation. However, rather than fully dismiss the anxiety, D deflects the question (turns 35–37: "I'd be quite interested to know what the neurosurgeons think," "I don't think I know," "what did he say?"). Once again, here there is a clear demarcation of expertise aimed at keeping genetic issues separate from neurosurgery. This is also an example of what Maynard (1991) referred to as perspective display sequence; that is, asking what else the clients know before formulating an expert opinion. It is clear that H was withholding the views of the neurosurgeon until asked (turn 36). In his assessment (turns 41 and 43), D foregrounds an information-giving frame, drawing on the functioning of membranes in an analytic way (see also Example 4 on skin patches). Talking about cells and membranes in a detached, scientific way allows for framing this as an information giving mode (turn 41–43, "you know . . . these membranes . . . have to grow . . ."). The expertise is evident in the description of how cells work and membranes grow and in the contrast suggested between a sore head caused by injury and the damage causing cells to divide and membranes to grow. In downplaying the extent of injury ("how can I put it," turn 43; "that sounds a bit unlikely," turn 45), D perhaps wants to reassure W about the inconsequentiality of the fall she suffered during her childhood.

The final excerpt presented here continues the interaction and signals the most critical moment in which clients choose to seek explicit advice. It is therefore necessary to reproduce this episode in full.

Example 7: Last resort

59 H: so it it eh- to cut a long story short (.) if eh your wife was in
        this position (God forbid) (.5) eh and you wanted another child
        would you say (.) the chances are so minute (.5) we can go
        ahead with one
        (.5)

60 H: ⌈it was your-

61 D: ⌊you're asking- (.) you're asking (.) two separate questions

62 H: if you were me or-

63 D: yeah=

64 H: =well yeah

65 D: but you're- you are asking two separate questions

66 H: mmh

67 D: you see there's the (.) the (.) the you know what you're saying
        one is (.) eh (.) is there a chance of eh (.) say of a child having
        a tendency to get meningiomas?
        (.5)

68 H: (unclear) (.) well I know I know it's like it would be the same
        chances as some (unclear)

69 D: yes that's very very unlikely

70 H: ⌈unlikely

71 D: ⌊so there's that question. and then there is the question of

72 H: mhm

73 D: of would the pregnancy cause another tumor
        (1.0)

74 D: and (.) I think the answer ⌈to that⌉=

75 H: ⌊that's ⌋(unclear)

76 D: =well I think (.) the pregnancy itself wouldn't cause another tumor (.) if there is a small recurrence eh that (.) was not identified on the scan (.) then I suppose a pregnancy could perhaps influence that rate of growth but (.) it's not going to make the difference between (.) the tumor coming back or not coming back (.5) it (.5) could make a (.) a difference to when it shows itself

77 H: mmh

78 D: but it would show itself anyway (.) but ehm:::

[few turns omitted where W and D talk about the arrangements for regular MRI scans]

79 W: I went to a CT scan (.) before this last year I went to a CT scan and MRI scan

80 D: yeah

81 W: and in CT scan I was sitting down in the waiting area and a woman (.) so we started chatting and eh- (.) so I thought well what's wrong with you you know there was nothing wrong with her face or anything she said I had meningioma (.) and it was- (.) it came here

82 D: right

83 W: and she said now it's eh come back after twelve years

84 D: ⌈right

85 H: ⌊mhm

          (1.0)

86 W: so she said eh (.) they can control it by medication and- (.)

87 D: yeah

88 W: because the registrar did tell me (.) they have a tendency coming back meningiomas=

89 H: =mhm

90 W: but when (.5) we don't know ⌈on the MRI scans

91 D: ⌊yeah yeah (.) yeah =yeah

92 H: yeah so- (.) it's eh=

93 W: =so it's all a matter of (.) luck (laughing)

94 H: yeah a shot in the dark shot in the dark you see (.5)

95 W/H: (laugh with sigh)

96 D: I think- (.) yeah. (.) I don't think a pregnancy is going to make the difference between a recurrence or not a recurrence

97 H: mmh (.)

98   D: yeah- (.) eh and eh (.) and there's no particular reason to
          think that you're more likely to have another- you know a
          separate tumor.=

99   W: =yeah, it's not eh (.) so much a matter of reoccurring (.) I
          mean <u>reoccurring</u> it's there whether I get pregnant or not isn't
          it? (.) it's <u>there</u>. ⌜it's only⌝ a matter=

100 D: ⌊yes   ⌋

101 W: =of ⌜<u>time</u> I guess when it's gonna show

102 D: ⌊yes   yes yes   yes=

103 W: =but pregnancy I think they eh meant it will speed up the (.)
          you know ⌜the process of it⌝ showing ⌜and-

104 D: ⌊but   ⌋   ⌊yeah
          (1.0)

105 D: but eh it's not so likely

106 W: it's not so likely

107 H: eh::::
          (.5)

108 D: I mean it's not so likely (.) you're not so very likely to have a
          recurrence anyway, because they <u>think</u> they removed it
          ⌜and the last

109 W: ⌊yeah I had two MRI scans and the result=

110 D: =the MRI scan ⌜was clear yeah ⌝

111 W: ⌊was okay but he⌟thought like within <u>two years</u>
          <u>if there is anything</u>

112 D: yeah

113 W: it will show on the MRI scan

114 D: yeah

115 W: and <u>then</u> we can (.) decide or give you the green light whether
          it's good to get pregnant or not

116 D: yeah

117 W: so (.) I don't know eh (.) in two years I (.) maybe I'll have a
          toddler running around (laughing) and we will decide what to
          do with a tumor (laughs)

118 H: (laughs)

119 D: =yeah (.) I - I - I - I don't think I can comment on

120 W: yeah

121 D: (.) on that. I mean I think that's something that the
          neurosurgeons are going to have a better

122   W: mmh
123   D: (.) or they can tell you better than I can (.)

With the formulation "to cut a long story short . . . ," H initiates role reversal in putting the doctor in the role of husband of W. In the genetic counseling context, a question such as "what would you do in my place" is considered "the famous–infamous question." Here it counts as a final attempt—similar to extreme case formulations for justifying intervention (Emerson, 1981)—by the clients at resolving the uncertainty. One underlying assumption is that D's preferred action script (in the role of husband to his wife with a tumor—God forbid!) would be a guide for the clients. Also, it amounts to casting D in the role of expert adviser as opposed to expert information giver. The delineation of his zone of (in)expertise thus assumes further significance in such moments, as it potentially offers a way out of a directed, advisory stance.

H's formulation resembles what Peräkylä (1995) would have called "hypothetical questioning," or what in Maynard's (1991) terms is a perspective display sequence (see D's use of this strategy in Example 6). Both Maynard and Peräkylä analyzed these discourse strategies as part of doctors' repertoire. Yet here we see that clients also selectively make use of such strategies to seek doctors' assessment prior to making up their minds. In his formulation "and you wanted another child" (turn 59), H is prefacing the fact that they are seriously thinking about another child. This is a last resort strategy for assessing the situation, and it also suggests that the discussion so far has been inconclusive. As with a perspective display sequence, which primarily serves as a face-saving mechanism, we can also see that such explicit advice-seeking routines prepare the ground for uncertainty reduction and therefore optimal uptake if expert advice were to be offered.

In turns 61–66, D can be seen as avoiding a direct response, a resistance to take up the role (either as "hypothetical husband" or as "expert adviser") created for him by H. However, it is arguable that he deliberately distances himself from giving a personal opinion or preference because in the context of this activity, a personal opinion is likely to be taken as a professional viewpoint.[8] The question posed by H is thus not taken up at that level. D instead revisits the entire purpose of the session, as he defines the concerns relating to the child having meningioma and W developing another tumor. D's remark in turn 65 ("you are asking two separate questions") frames a further information-giving sequence—as a form of expertise in terms of risk calculation in relation to another pregnancy. H's question about whether or not W should try for another pregnancy is thus deflected as he goes over information more explicitly (see Sarangi, 2000a, for a detailed analysis of this fragment in terms of information-as-explanation sequence). Underlying this is a shift from H's question about decision making as partners and potential parents (whether or not to have a pregnancy) to an objectified discussion of risks about the tumor coming back or not coming back.[9] Rather than refute the request directly, D rephrases it to be able to provide more information rather than advice, which amounts to signaling a possible miscommunication of information already provided.[10]

W initiates another information-giving sequence in a narrative form (turn 81 and following). Both these narratives, however, act as volunteering of additional information with the hope of pushing the expert toward formulation of a clear and certain standpoint. Unlike the previous occasion (see Example 6) in which W narrates the head injury she had sustained in her childhood and the possibility of that contributing to the recurrence or development of a tumor, this time she offers more pressing evidence (recurrence of a tumor in the case of another person) and foregrounds her discomfort at the scan results. In saying "and she said now it's eh come back after twelve years" (turn 83), W can be heard as generalizing from evidence from other people. In turn 88, W substantiates her view by recruiting the expert voice of the registrar ("because the registrar did tell me (.) they have a tendency coming back meningiomas"). Note that W is using an objectification strategy typical of expert talk by personifying meningiomas as "they"—which can be talked about independent of people affected by them.

In turn 96, D once again reiterates his expert knowledge-giving role as opposed to expert advice-giving role. He seems to be more definitive than before in suggesting that pregnancy is not a risk factor. We can see this as a form of reassurance but interspersed with an element of uncertainty. This is followed by a disagreement sequence. D is once again taking the scan as the evidence for formulating his opinion. Consider his following remarks:

"I don't think a pregnancy is going to make the difference between a recurrence or not a recurrence" (turn 96).

"You're not so very likely to have a recurrence anyway, because they think they removed it" (turn 108).

We can see a link between these two pronouncements. If the tumor has been removed and the MRI scan does not show any trace, then the issue of recurrence is not relevant. Whether pregnancy will cause another tumor is a matter that falls outside the expertise of D here, as can be seen later (turn 119 and following). Between turns 99 and 103, W displays her understanding of what counts as certain (the tumor is there) and what counts as uncertain (the time when it's going to show and that pregnancy will trigger the pace). In turn 117, W poses the question not just in terms of a dilemma ("to get pregnant or not," turn 115), but more as a possible reality ("maybe I'll have a toddler running around . . . and we will decide what to do with a tumor"). D finally withdraws from this stage of decision making (turns 119–123), and he does so once again by deflecting expert opinion to the neurosurgeons. Implicitly, perhaps, D gives "the green light."

CONCLUSION: THE ETHOS OF
NONDIRECTIVENESS

In our analysis we have focused specifically on the interplay of different discourse strategies that genetic counselors can draw on to strike a balance between affirming their zone of expertise (mainly through contrast devices) and disclaiming sufficient knowledge in adjacent fields of knowledge. Such a framing allows them to formulate uncertainty (mainly through hedging devices) without risking their authority, as well as avoiding taking on the role of an expert adviser.

One can advance various reasons for why the geneticist does not usually play the part that might be expected but instead deflects authority to the neurosurgeon. To begin with, as we have seen, there may be genuine uncertainty in relation to the information sought by the clients—that is, what might be the precise link between pregnancy and recurrence of a tumor. Although the clients may have formulated their questions as a search for "facts," the facts may not be known, and facts alone might not fully answer their underlying concerns. There may also be a wider family dimension to be considered by the counselor, including issues relating to personal relationships or emotional responses to a situation. In other words, the client cannot be considered in isolation. It is equally conceivable that the professionals are operating with a fear of possible litigation or of undermining clients' strongly held principles or convictions such as ethical positions or religious beliefs. Finally, and more important, the ethos of genetic counseling is heavily influenced by adherence to the slogan of nondirectiveness. The emphasis on nondirectiveness in genetic counseling serves important functions for the professionals in addition to its use in the management of uncertainty. The explicit handing of all responsibility for decisions about genetic testing and reproductive issues to their clients helps the counselors in two important respects: (a) it makes their work emotionally easier through discouraging overinvolvement with clients and by ensuring what Elwyn, Gray, and Clarke (2000) called *shared decision making*; and (b) it simplifies the legal responsibility for client decisions, making it more difficult for clients to sue professionals if the outcome is in some way unsatisfactory.

The combination of uncertainty inherent in the discipline and the adherence of clinical genetics professionals to nondirectiveness has a major impact on the nature of the genetic counseling clinic. Not only does the clinical geneticist have to acknowledge the uncertainty that is such a feature of this professional field, but he or she is also expected not to give advice to clients. One consequence is that the authority of the clinical geneticist may not be so readily apparent to clients. Both factors could seem likely to undermine the professional's authority as an expert; therefore, the professionals' efforts to enhance the credibility of their professional role in the face of lingering uncertainty and their reluctance to give advice make the negotiation of the expert–lay relationship a most complex topic.

NOTES

1 Wolff and Jung (1995) characterized genetic counseling as "information about information." This would mean that counseling involves an evaluation of what patients already have as information and what new information the counselor chooses to provide.

2 In genetic clinics dealing with the polycystic kidney disease condition, a kidney specialist is often present. The interaction then reflects the division of labor between the geneticist and the kidney specialist.

3 According to Hewitt and Stokes (1975), disclaimers function prospectively in contrast to accounts (Scott & Lyman, 1968) that function retrospectively. It is, however, difficult to maintain such a temporal distinction.

4 Hopper et al. (1995) suggested that embedded disclaimers are common in information-giving sequences.

5 The following symbols differ from the journal's transcription default system: dots or numerical values between round brackets denote pause, texts within double round brackets are glosses, square brackets signal overlaps, and untranscribable segments are signaled by [^^^^^]. The line numbers refer to the main transcript, but for purposes of analysis of individual examples we use turn numbers.

6 In this instance, W and H decline the offer of a physical examination.

7 What has gone before, especially when D expands on how genes work, can be seen as information exchange sequences with a display of expert knowledge.

8 This is perhaps the opposite of what Jefferson and Lee (1981) said about potential "rejection of advice" when it is offered in response to unfolding "troubles talk."

9 This can be regarded as a stance of neutrality, as the topic of the second pregnancy becomes backgrounded. Such neutrality is observable in divorce mediation settings in which counselors refrain from commenting on certain aspects of partners' relationships as they focus on parental responsibilities and rights over children in question (Greatbatch & Dingwall, 1999).

10 D here can be seen as rehearsing A/B events in Labov and Fanshel's (1977) terms (see Sarangi, 2000b).

REFERENCES

Atkinson, P. (1995). *Medical talk and medical work.* London: Sage.

Atkinson, P. (1999). Medical discourse, evidentiality and the construction of professional responsibility. In S. Sarangi & C. Roberts (Eds.), *Talk, work and institutional order: Discourse in medical, mediation and management settings* (pp. 75–107). Berlin, Germany: Mouton de Gruyter.

Bauman, Z. (1993). *Postmodern ethics.* Oxford, England: Blackwell.

Beach, W. A., & Metzger, T. R. (1997). Claiming insufficient knowledge. *Human Communication Research, 23,* 562–588.

Beck, U. (1992). *Risk society: Towards a new modernity.* London: Sage.

Candlin, C. N., & Lucas, J. (1986). Interpretations and explanations in discourse: Modes of "advising" in family planning. In T. Ensink, A. van Essen, & T. van der Geest (Eds.), *Discourse analysis and public life* (pp. 13–38). Dordrecht, The Netherlands: Foris.

Clarke, A. (1991). Is non-directive genetic counseling possible? *Lancet, 338,* 998–1001.

Clarke, A. (1997). The process of genetic counseling: Beyond non-directiveness. In P. S. Harper & A. J. Clarke (Eds.), *Genetics, society and clinical practice* (pp. 179–200). Oxford, England: Bios Scientific.

Douglas, M. (1986). *Risk acceptability according to the social sciences.* London: Routledge & Kegan Paul.

Douglas, M. (1990). Risk as a forensic resource. *Daedalus, 119*(4), 1–16.

Douglas, M. (1992). *Risk and blame: Essays in cultural theory.* London: Routledge.

Dubois, B. L. (1987). "Something on the order of around forty to forty four": Imprecise numerical expressions in biomedical slide talks. *Language in Society, 16,* 527–541.

Elwyn, G. J., Gray, J., & Clarke, A. J. (2000). Shared decision making and non-directiveness in genetic counseling. *Journal of Medical Genetics, 37,* 135–138.

Emerson, R. M. (1981). On last resorts. *American Journal of Sociology, 87,* 1–22.

Fox, R. (1957). Training for uncertainty. In R. K. Merton, G. G. Reader, & P. L. Kendall (Eds.), *The student physician: Introductory studies in the sociology of medical education* (pp. 207–241). Cambridge, MA: Harvard University Press.

Goodwin, C. (1994). Professional vision. *American Anthropologist, 96,* 606–633.

Greatbatch, D., & Dingwall, R. (1999). Professional neutralism in family mediation. In S. Sarangi & C. Roberts (Eds.), *Talk, work and institutional order: Discourse in medical, mediation and management settings* (pp. 271–292). Berlin, Germany: Mouton de Gruyter.

Hacking, I. (1975). *The emergence of probability.* Cambridge, England: Cambridge University Press.

Hewitt, J. P., & Stokes, R. (1975). Disclaimer. *American Sociological Review, 40,* 1–11.

Hopper, R., Ward, J. A., Thomason, W. R., & Sias, P. M. (1995). Two types of institutional disclaimers at the Cancer Information Service. In G. H. Morris & R. J. Chenail (Eds.), *The talk of the clinic: Explorations in the analysis of medical and therapeutic discourse* (pp. 171–184). Mahwah, NJ: Lawrence Erlbaum Associates, Inc.

Hughes, E. (1981). *Men and their work.* Westport, CT: Greenwood. (Original work published 1958)

Jefferson, G., & Lee, J. R. E. (1981). The rejection of advice: Managing the problematic convergence of a "troubles-telling" and a "service encounter." *Journal of Pragmatics, 5,* 399–422.

Johnson, R. H., & Blair, J. A. (1983). *Logical self-defense* (2nd ed.). Toronto: McGraw-Hill Ryerson.

Labov, W., & Fanshel, D. (1977). *Therapeutic discourse: Psychotherapy as conversation.* New York: Academic.

Luhmann, N. (1993). *Risk: A sociological theory* (R. Barrett, Trans.). New York: Aldine de Gruyter.

Maynard, D. W. (1991). The perspective-display series and the delivery and receipt of diagnostic news. In D. Boden & D. Zimmerman (Eds.), *Talk and social structure* (pp. 164–192). Cambridge, England: Polity.

Michie, S., Bron, F., Bobrow, M., & Marteau, T. M. (1997). Nondirectiveness in genetic counseling: An empirical study. *American Journal of Human Genetics, 60,* 40–47.

Mishler, E. G. (1984). *The discourse of medicine: Dialectics of medical interviews.* Norwood, NJ: Ablex.

Parsons, E., & Atkinson, P. (1992). Lay constructions of genetic risks. *Sociology of Health and Illness, 14,* 437–455.

Parsons, E., & Atkinson, P. (1993). Genetics risk and reproduction. *The Sociological Review, 41,* 679–706.

Peräkylä, A. (1995). *AIDS counseling: Institutional interaction and clinical practice.* Cambridge, England: Cambridge University Press.

Pomerantz, A. (1984). Agreeing and disagreeing with assessments: Some features of preferred/dispreferred turn shapes. In J. M. Atkinson & J. Heritage (Eds.), *Structures of social action: Studies in conversation analysis* (pp. 152–163). Cambridge, England: Cambridge University Press.

Prince, E. F., Frader, J., & Bosk, C. (1982). On hedging in physician–physician discourse. In R. di Pietro (Ed.), *Linguistics and the professions* (pp. 83–97). Norwood, NJ: Ablex.

Sarangi, S. (2000a). Activity types, discourse types and interactional hybridity: The case of genetic counseling. In S. Sarangi & M. Coulthard (Eds.), *Discourse and social life* (pp. 1–27). London: Pearson.

Sarangi, S. (2000b, May). *Narratives of uncertainty: Managing A/B events in genetic counseling.* Paper presented at the Conference on European Worldview: Narratives of European Life, La Londe-les Maures, France.

Sarangi, S. (2002). The language of likelihood in genetic counseling discourse. *Journal of Language and Social Psychology, 21,* 7–31.

Sarangi, S., & Clarke, A. J. (2002). Constructing an account by contrast in counseling for childhood genetic testing. *Social Science & Medicine, 54,* 295–308.

Sarangi, S., & Roberts, C. (Eds.). (1999). *Talk, work and institutional order: Discourse in medical, mediation and management settings.* Berlin, Germany: Mouton de Gruyter.

Schutz, A. (1964). *Collected papers* (Vol. 2). Hague, The Netherlands: Nijhoff.

Scott, M., & Lyman, S. (1968). Accounts. *American Sociological Review, 33,* 46–62.

Silverman, D. (1987). *Communication and medical practice: Social relations in the clinic.* London: Sage.

Silverman, D. (1997). *Discourses of counseling: HIV counseling as social interaction.* London: Sage.

van Zuuren, F. J., van Schie, E. C. M., & van Baaren, N. K. (1997). Uncertainty in the information provided during genetic counseling. *Patient Education and Counseling, 32,* 129–139.

Wachtel, T. (1980). Pragmatic approximations. *Journal of Pragmatics, 4,* 201–211.

Williams, S., & Calnan, M. (1996). Modern medicine and the lay populace: Theoretical perspectives and methodological issues. In S. Williams & M. Calnan (Eds.), *Modern medicine: Lay perspectives and experiences* (pp. 2–25). London: UCL Press.

Wolff, G., & Jung, C. (1995). Nondirectiveness and genetic counseling. *Journal of Genetic Counseling, 4,* 3–25.

APPENDIX
OVERALL TRACKING OF THE
DELINEATION OF (IN)EXPERTISE

Line Numbers (in transcript)	Initiation and Scope
10–13	H explains that referral was from neurosurgeon.
39–41	W reports how neurosurgeon stated that he was not the best person to answer questions about pregnancies and maternal age (and also perhaps about a tumor).
41–49	W points to the conflicting advice from two neurosurgeons and GP about wisdom of a pregnancy—so GP referred them to genetics.
50–61	H goes over the risk of recurrence of the original tumor—surgeon thinks it's all out but can't be certain. (This account is reinforced by W in lines 62–68.)
82–86	W reports GP's opinion regarding the decision about timing of Clomid—that it should await genetics consultation.
92–94	W did not want home visit by genetics team because they (the family) know condition is not hereditary.
113–115	D respecifies the question: "You were at risk of the meningioma recurring."
138–140	W wants to know if a pregnancy would put her health at risk.
144–152	D outlines his own interpretation of what the referral is about and once again attempts to respecify the scope of the discussion—"the likely influence of pregnancy on [pace of] recurrence."
175–186	D offers an assessment of the linkage between pregnancy and recurrence; he supports this assessment on the evidence that "the MRI scan has been normal" (in the same way that H and W see the scan as normal; D disclaims any further expertise "I'm not in a good position to advise . . . the neurosurgeons . . . have a much better idea."
249–256; 265–266	D reiterates his position: "It's just not my field really . . . the opinions of the neurosurgeons would make more sense."
287–297	D tries to steer the discussion in the direction of his expertise—"the sort of question I had thought . . . you'd be bringing to me [discussion of D's ideas about domain of clinical genetics and purpose of home visit by genetics nurse].
360 and following	General discussion about whether D needs to examine W to look for skin marks—but they know her body well enough so that this is not needed.
365–375	D explicitly demarcates areas where he can make statements and areas where he cannot.
403–411	H cites research indicating meningiomas may be caused by head injuries.
422–423	D once again defers any expert opinion: "I'd be quite interested to know what the neurosurgeons think [about the head injury issue]."

(Continued)

Line Numbers *(in transcript)*	Initiation and Scope
537–541	W reports neurosurgeon's view: "he thought like within two years if there is anything it will show on the MRI scan. . . ."
542–545	D distances himself: "I don't think I can comment on that . . . the neurosurgeons. . . ."
547–549	W points to contradicting expert opinions: "The main surgeon . . . comes up with one opinion and then this one comes up with another."
556–570	W continues with how the neurosurgeon is contradicted by cosmetic surgeon: So—"I think each one speaks within their field you know."
581–584	W reports the surgeon's view: "No it's after thirty-five they say you have to have more tests . . ." [appeal to "they" as common knowledge].
614–615	D finally declines any further assessment of the situation: "But I just know some of the things you're asking it's really for the neurosurgeons to say."
626	H makes the point about confusion arising from conflicting advice.

Note.   H = husband; W = wife; GP = general practitioner; D = geneticist.

Research on Language and Social Interaction, 35(2), 173–193

Taking Risks: An Indicator of Expertise?

Sally Candlin
Department of Nursing, Family and Community Health
University of Western Sydney, New South Wales

The achievement of excellence in nursing practice is reflected in the quality of the nurse's discourse. The identifying features of expertise in nurse–patient discourse relate to the ability to construct a coherent text in which the power relations are negotiated between nurse and patient. Data were drawn from nurse–patient interactions using a nursing assessment proforma. In this instance the instrument is used as a means of investigating discourse strategies. The nurses are an experienced registered nurse delivering care to clients in their homes in the community and a nurse who has no formal nursing qualifications but works as an assistant in nursing in an aged-care residential facility (nursing home). The strategies employed involve the expert nurse risking that the interaction will become a social, rather than a therapeutic interaction. An analysis of the texts demonstrates that the interaction between the expert nurse and the patient is rich in appropriate and pertinent information, providing a sound basis for appropriate nursing care. Both expert nurse and patient expand topics so that the health advice given is appropriate to the meaning to the patient of the health situation. This contrasts with the untrained nurse, who is found to control topic management and to disallow patient digressions. Such a conversation cannot be regarded as either a therapeutic interaction or a rich social interaction.

Aged care is considered by some, and often at the policy-making level, to constitute "basic" nursing care, the implication being that the required level of care does not of necessity demand the skills of experienced

Correspondence concerning this article should be sent to Sally Candlin, Department of Nursing, Family, and Community Health, University of Western Sydney, NSW, Australia. E-mail: scandlin@ozemail.com.au and highly educated nurses. In-depth discussion of the ideology on which this stance is based is not the focus of this article, neither is it the purpose of this article to discuss the various types of health care delivery systems as they pertain to aged care. What is important to acknowledge is that much of the "hands-on" care in many aged-care facilities in Western countries is given by staff who sometimes have no formal nursing qualifications. The argument underpinning this work is that geriatric nursing care is the most complex form of care and makes heavy demands on the expertise of nurses. I argue that direct care of older people should be given by experienced nurses who are trained to manage effectively the strategies required to engage in therapeutic communication—that is, communication that contributes to the healing process, recognizing that healing is multidimensional: physical, psychological, social, spiritual, and emotional.

To demonstrate the differences in expertise, examining the professional discourse practices of different levels of nurse and the outcomes of those practices is central. Nursing care is not only characteristically mediated through discourse, but the nature of its quality is dependent on sensitive discourse practices. This article is based on a study conducted by the author and considered the care given by different levels of nurses in different settings. The majority of older people in Western countries live in their homes in the community, often supported by health or welfare services, or both, and frequently including the care of registered nurses (RNs) who are community based. However, approximately 7% of people over the age of 65 years need to be cared for in residential aged-care facilities where care is often given by staff with no formal qualifications but supervised by RNs.

The participants in the data drawn on in this article were two nurses, representative of a larger study (Candlin, 1997) involving 30 nurse–patient dyads. One of the nurses was an RN based in the community who was discussing the health needs of an older woman whom she had previously visited. The second nurse, who was not an RN, was employed in an aged-care facility and was discussing the health needs of an older female resident known to her.

Numerous activities constitute nursing practice, not least of which is the assessment of the patient's nursing and health needs. In such situations, information about one member of the nurse–patient dyad (the patient) must be elicited by the other (the nurse). The reverse rarely happens. Although Rogers (1967) suggested that there is mutuality in the professional relationship (between the helper and the one being helped), Morrison (1994) cited

Buber (1966), who argued the contrary, suggesting that because the patient comes to the professional for help there can be no mutuality. The nurse–patient relationship, particularly as it is demonstrated in the situations described here, reflects this lack of mutuality. The situations may be considered demanding because they rely solely on observations and communicative skills. This type of assessment does not involve the use of clinical instruments (e.g., blood pressure measuring equipment) and physical assessment such as auscultation and palpation. Rather it is the eliciting of verbal information based on a proforma that covers numerous topic areas (e.g., previous health history, degree and nature of mobility, dental care, diet, hygiene, social support, hearing, vision, and psychological state). The information-gathering process, however, is unique to each situation because there may be occasions in which some information is already known, and eliciting it is considered to be inappropriate at that particular moment.

Although both nurses considered here knew the patient with whom they were interacting, neither nurse had previously used the particular proforma. Although the nursing assistant (N2) was not expected to be familiar with assessment procedures per se, all nurses were, and are, expected to demonstrate communicative competence. The nurses were told by the researcher that the proforma was to be used as a trigger for generating communication between patient and nurse and were advised to familiarize themselves with the topics by doing "dummy runs" until they were confident about the process. They were advised that if the conversation sidetracked and a topic was mentioned that occurred later in the proforma, then they should be flexible and allow such digressions, not necessarily following strictly the given order of topics. This was to encourage the eliciting of information that was meaningful to the patient. Such advice was particularly pertinent for nurses who were unaccustomed to assessing health needs, as in the case of untrained or inexperienced staff (such as N2). This approach is supported by the work of Faulkner (1992), who argued that the nurse directing and asking questions does not necessarily result in the gathering of rich information. Faulkner's argument is that when a nurse is prepared to allow the patient to talk, the patient will usually discuss what is meaningful and important to him or her rather than being guided into talking about topics that present no problem and are perceived to be unimportant. One knows that to handle such situations demands experience on the part of the nurse, and this is a later focus in the article.

Underpinning the current practice of many health workers is an overall philosophy guiding the principles of primary health care in which the patient is encouraged to be a coworker in the needs identification process and in consequent goal setting, enabling the patient to be self-determining in the decision-making process. However, an accurate assessment demands that in this process the patient disclose information that may be considered to be embarrassing and face threatening to the patient. Accordingly, the assessment process must develop a trusting professional relationship between nurse and patient so that the interaction is not a simple friendly social interaction but becomes one that is therapeutic. As such, the focus is directed at the discoursal choices the participants make to achieve nursing goals. These choices have the potential to impose a degree of risk: a concept that implies danger, chance, and at best uncertainty. In assessment situations in which face is threatened, the risk that the nurse takes in encouraging autonomous or shared decision making is that the patient will not disclose essential information, which may result in less than accurate assessments and consequently less than adequate care. The risk in this situation is not, therefore, one of developing disease per se. Rather it is the risk that is undertaken daily in normal conversations: the risk of being misunderstood, the risk of losing face. In the nurse–patient assessment situation, however, there is the added risk of leaving unsaid what should be said. I am not therefore referring here to statistical risk ratios or multiple risk factors but, nevertheless, very real risks to health if erroneous decisions are made and inappropriate health-related advice is given on the basis of inaccurate or insufficient information. In this article I address the notion of risk and uncertainty as it relates to discoursal choices in accomplishing the nursing assessment of a person's health status, that is, his or her state of health. What are the strategic adjustments that interlocutors need to make to minimize the risk of making a less than adequate assessment? What are the risks taken by the patient and the nurse?

IDENTIFYING DISCOURSAL STRATEGIES IN ASSESSMENT SITUATIONS

I begin by concentrating on two pragmatic features that the nurse draws on to perform an accurate and comprehensive health assessment, the successful completion of which identifies her as an expert nurse (cf. Benner, 1984). Because assessment covers many areas, topic management is one such feature. Because topic management is closely connected with the framing of the activity, it makes sense to compare the different framings adopted in two situations. The effectiveness of topic management is in turn closely linked with the notion of coherence, the achievement of which is not simple when performing a comprehensive and multidimensional health assessment covering social, physical, emotional, psychological, and spiritual needs. Data, however, demonstrate that coherence is achievable, and assessments can be thorough and accurate if the nurse adopts certain strategies relating to these pragmatic features.

Framing in Assessment Situations

How the nurse introduces and frames the interaction is crucial to the ultimate success of both the professional relationship and the achievement of goals because the frame constitutes the "instructions which a speaker gives to the listener on how to understand the discourse message" (Ribeiro, 1996, p. 182). The initial framing of the interaction provides the basis for its conduct, but this may be open to misinterpretation because, as Jones (1996) asserted, "when we speak we never speak the same language. We engage in a discourse system made up of rules and expectations and ways of seeing the world which we take for granted" (p. 2). Ways of seeing the world are culturally defined and if the interlocutor from a different speech community attributes attitudes, aims, and meaning that the speaker does not intend, then the interaction may be open to misunderstanding and ultimately is at risk of breaking down.

Briggs (1986) argued that when establishing a referential frame, "reference is both a creative and a powerful act, as it provides an inter-subjective link between speaker and hearer" (p. 51). He continued: "One or more entities, processes, imaginative constructions, and so on are selected by the speaker from an infinitude of referential possibilities, and are re-created in the mind of the hearer" (p. 51). In making reference to Garfinkel's (1967) argument that utterances are frequently vague, Briggs's "re-creation" can always then be only approximate. Questions must be posed that are not only clear but possess such specificity that make them unambiguous to the hearer. The frame needs to indicate the speaker's intent so the interlocutor understands the discourse message and can work within the same frame. Without this clarity and understanding there is risk, not only of communication breakdown, but of a consequent inadequate or incomplete assessment affecting goals, nursing interventions, and outcomes.

The nurse needs to recognize the patient's past experiences in the framing of the event and his or her subsequent discoursal attitudes and behaviors because topics in assessment situations may relate to the presentation of self and the individual's values and belief systems. Within the frame, speakers must not only be aware of the understanding and expectations of their interlocutors but also of the alignments that each takes within the interaction (cf. Goffman, 1974). The frame thus becomes an indicator of how the discourse is expected to proceed, and sets boundaries on the relationship. In Example 1, the RN (N1) frames the assessment as a conversation in which the talk is going to be about the patient (Mrs. C). This is in contrast to Example 2 in which the non-RN (N2) frames the activity as an interview.

Example 1

```
01   N1:   thank you for taking part in this research today.
02          we're just going to be talking about you (3) and how
03          you manage at home that sort of thing we've been
04          coming to you for some months now haven't we
```

Example 2

```
01   N2:   . . . and I'm going to interview you if you don't mind
2           on a few questions about yourself
```

It is interesting that the event framed as an interview is conducted by a non-RN, whereas the RN uses a conversational frame. The second patient, Mrs. B, who is being assessed by the non-RN, N2, is to understand that the interaction will take the form of an interview in which the interviewee will have little control over the items to be addressed. It is the nurse who will take control and who knows the questions. Mrs. B will have little control; indeed she is not expected to know the questions or the rules of "the game." In determining the nature and process of the interaction, N2 avoids the risk of allowing Mrs. B to control the conversation. It is assumed that knowledge of the regulative and constitutive rules that govern interview situations is known by each participant. From a discourse organizational viewpoint, Mrs. B is not consciously involved in the task of assessment.

In contrast, Mrs. C in Example 1, who is being assessed by an RN, understands that they are "just going to be talking," where the informality implies that both participants have equal control over the interaction. Furthermore, the mitigating "just," in line 2, suggests that this is not a formidable procedure but one that should be free of stress and an occasion in which both can be relaxed and informal. N1, however, is taking a risk. She risks Mrs. C taking control and raising questions that may be unrelated to the assessment activity. The different degrees of risk taking remain appropriate to the situation and the availability of members' resources (cf. Fairclough, 1989)—that is, the particular resources available to the individual by virtue of education, training, experience, position, and authority within the institution. Following Bourdieu (1991, 1993), and in particular his discussion of educational "capital," N1 has greater capital on which to draw. As such she can afford to take greater risks, but as an RN she also has greater obligations in that she is held responsible for her nursing interventions. To intervene appropriately she needs to draw from Mrs. C as much information as possible. N1 therefore encourages the disclosure of information, and to accomplish this she must establish a considerable degree of trust. She places herself in a cost–benefit situation. The cost to N1 is the risk that Mrs. C will take charge and demand more of her member's resources of her capital than she has available. The potential benefit is that the trust engendered by the empowerment of Mrs. C as an equal partner in the interaction will facilitate rich disclosure of information beneficial to achieving her nursing goals.

Topic Management

When examining the data in the following Examples 3 and 4, it becomes clear that the assessment proforma is being used by N2 to gather only itemized information. The information is gathered in the order in which the items appear on the proforma and as they are raised only by the nurse. This may be because the nurse is unfamiliar with the proforma and is unaccustomed to administering nursing assessments, or because she, the nurse, expects that she should control the situation and thus selects the topics that are defined by the institution. For N2 then, in choosing to frame the event as an interview, the order of the topics becomes predetermined. No scope is allowed for digressions that might trigger other topics or allow a topic to be discussed from different perspectives, even though these might produce more information (see Example 3, lines 1, 2, 7). (Note in Example 3 that there is no expansion of the topic that might have further explored the adequacy of dentures and the link to an adequate diet.) The patient relinquished control to the participant perceived as having more power.

Example 3

01	N2:	and your hygiene well that's very good
02		a very clean person (3) em your teeth
03		they your own teeth (3)
04	Mrs. B:	no
05		they're false
06	N2:	hh(2) dentures dentures right (6) and
07		your diet's good isn't it

In Example 4, in contrast, N1 elects to conduct the assessment as a conversation giving opportunity for digressions that might then trigger other topics (see the contribution of Mrs. C in Example 4, lines 9, 11, 18, and 19). However, the inherent risk is that amount of information would then need to be processed and would present her with a formidable task. Not only would she need to sift the relevant from the irrelevant information, but she would also need to retain the relevant information to add to the accumulating data on that particular assessment topic.

Example 4: N1 and Mrs. C

01	N1:	thank you for taking part in this research today
02		we're just going to be talking about you (3) and
03		how you manage at home that sort of thing we've
04		been coming to you for some months now
05		haven't we
06	Mrs. C:	yes
07	N1:	helping you with your showering you're starting to
08		feel better about that now aren't you
09	Mrs. C:	oh yes feeling more confident too
10	N1:	mm that's good
11	Mrs. C:	but as I say you know if I didn't feel well and I was ( )
12		I wouldn't have=
13		=you're sure that there's a nice support

```
14              in that shower with the rail and all that in it
15  Mrs. C:    yes
16  N1:        and the rubber mat now that you've got=
17  Mrs. C:    =my stick has
18              been in the kitchen for two days not used=
19              =right so
20              you're becoming stronger ⌐that's⌐ good isn't it
21  Mrs. C:                              ⌊ yes ⌋
22              I nearly had a little slip in the bathroom last night I tell
23              you what I did in the bathroom one ⌐nigh⌐t before I go to bed
24  N1:                                            ⌊mm⌋
25  Mrs. C:    I might go to bed about half past five or something like that
26              but I put the light on in the bathroom all night and the first
27              time I turn it off is when I get up in the morn⌐ing⌐
28  N1:                                                     ⌊tha⌋t's a
29              good idea isn't it just gives you a bit of light around
30  Mrs. C:    yes and it gives me a little bit of confidence
```

The discourse in the conversational frame proceeds quickly, demonstrated by the latching of utterances between speakers and the overlapping utterances as the nurse takes every opportunity to encourage and show approval by aligning with the patient—for example, lines 3 to 14, 20, and 29 (cf. Goffman, 1967). The conversation flows easily from one topic to another, enabling them to be addressed from different perspectives. Starting with the assessment topic of hygiene (showering), it then shifts to confidence (lack of which often appears to result from illness or trauma), which in turn shifts to safety: support, bath mat, and stick (the latter indicating a level of mobility). The amount of information gleaned for each topic addressed provides an index of a rich and in-depth assessment. What is also interesting to note is that N1 is seen almost to make a false start in her first utterance (lines 1–5) in which she attempts to establish a conversational frame, resulting in a monosyllabic answer "yes." It seems that there was insufficient information for Mrs. C to maintain the conversational frame until N1 gave further "information" (cf. Ribeiro, 1999). N1's rapid strategic adjustment facilitated Mrs. C's understanding of the requirements of the event, which allowed her to volunteer information before questions were asked. This enabled her to establish her power base in the interaction because she chose what and how much information she wished to disclose. The resulting coherence in this discourse stems from more than just the structuring provided by the proforma. Later in the interaction, N1 refers back to previous discourse topics (in Example 6, following, she is seen to refer back to the stick and mobility that first appeared in Example 4). Such cross-referencing is not simply facilitating coherent discourse; it expands the discussion of the topic of *mobility*. N1 is making the topic meaningful for Mrs. C in the way that she links *mobility* to *confidence, hygiene,* and *safety* in Example 4; *social activities* in Example 6; and *shopping* and *diet* in Example 7 when Mrs. C volunteered "now I haven't been to see the butcher since March." This is in contrast to the evidence presented in the assessment of Mrs. B by N2 in which she appeared to be closely bound by the structure of the proforma. *Mobility* was not discussed except to state "you're bed bound now aren't you" and "no outdoor ability." When Mrs. B responded "unfortunately," this response was not developed. Similarly, a question by N2 relating to hearing was not developed following the acknowledgment that the person was deaf. N2 appears not to make hearing impairment meaningful for the patient by not relating to social activities or by not discussing a hearing aid.

The concept of coherence must be addressed in more depth to determine the strategies that are used to achieve discourse that both maintains the conversational frame while addressing multiple topics and at the same time makes meaning from seemingly disparate topics such that appropriate advice may be given.

Coherence

In each of the assessments from which the preceding data are taken, the interactions involving N1 and N2 might be judged to be coherent if only because each has as its focus the health of the patient. Intuitively, however, one might perceive one interaction to be more coherent than the other. For example, the data reveal that topics in which a question–answer (interview) approach is adopted appear to have no particular link with each other or with any other topic in the discourse. The only link between the topics is that they appear as items on the proforma. All of the utterances are determined by the assessment items and occur in the order given. Such coherence stems only from the overriding purpose of the interaction, and is driven by the instrument employed. This coherence will be termed *simple coherence.* In contrast, where topics under discussion do not appear in any set order—the discourse taking the form of an informal conversation—one topic appears to provide a cue for the introduction of another. (This, of course, is not dissimilar from the argument presented by Jefferson [1984, p. 198] in her discussion of step-wise transition in troubles telling.) The coherence demonstrated within such discourse will be referred to as *comprehensive coherence*. This coherence is dependent on skillful topic management but more than this also demonstrates expert nursing care in the way that it furthers the understanding by the nurse of the depth to which she must probe to elicit the level of understanding of the patient of the significance of possible functional deficits.

Comprehensive coherence: The appearance of strands.   Analysis of the text produced by N1 and Mrs. C suggests that not only are numerous assessment topic items addressed to be found in the proforma, but there are also recurring elements or themes that appear as "strands" running through the whole text. These strands are distinct from the topic items introduced in the proforma. They are best regarded as discourse topics raised in the conversation, often in relation to assessment topic items, and that appear to direct and shape the discourse. They thus have a discoursal function. At other times, they are topics introduced spontaneously by either interlocutor. Strands provide the main themes because they recur throughout the text and simultaneously display semantic and discoursal functions, helping to shape the discourse and provide a measure of its coherence. For example, in contrast to the discourse of N1 and Mrs. C in which three strands are identified, only one strand can be identified in the discourse of N2 and Mrs. B, which appears not to play a vital semantic and discoursal role, neither shaping nor giving long-term direction to the interaction.

Goffman (1974, p. 210) referred to the notion of "attentional tracks," proposing that within any social encounter there is activity that moves the event further along. This activity is within the "main line" or "storyline track" and is germane to the successful understanding of the event by both participants. Storyline tracks can be seen to be vital in establishing and maintaining the assessment within the nursing activity. The three strands in the assessment of Mrs. C provide an interactional structure, evidencing their discoursal role. We can identify these strands as *time, confidence,* and *progress.* They are introduced in the first exchanges as seen in Example 4.

The first strand appears in line 4 in the nurse's first utterance, "we've been coming to you for <u>some months</u> now" (Strand 1, *time*). Here it can be seen that two lexical items ("months" and "now") are semantically linked and collocate in a lexical phrase signifying the notion of duration of time. There is an indication that the situation is ongoing, linking, in this example, the past to the present ("we've been coming" and "now"). The second strand appears in line 9 (Mrs. C's second turn) when Mrs. C says "oh yes feeling more confident too" (Strand 2, *confidence*). The lexical item "confidence" recurs throughout the discourse and is known by health professionals to be an indicator of improved health. N1 recognizes that confidence is an important factor to Mrs. C in determining her restoration to health and normal functioning. She thus aligns with the nursing role in delivering patient care and identifies the development of patient confidence as one of the criteria for the achievement of goals. Confidence is also linked with the *progress* strand that is introduced in line 20, "right so you're becoming stronger [that's] good" (Strand 3, *progress*). This strand is indicated by the morphological element "er" and is linked with the process verb "becoming." It denotes an ongoing situation and as such links with the strand *time* and the notion of linking past with present and future. As we indicated, this strand is also related to that of *confidence*.

Note that the "informal talk" frame is being maintained as the three strands are being initiated and the first two assessment topics introduced, all taking place within the first four exchanges. The discourse in lines 22–24 references "time" in each line, with "night" being mentioned three times. Similarly the mention of "light" in line 25 (and its reference "it" in line 26) is picked up by N1 in line 28 and again by Mrs. C in line 30 when she says, "it gives me a little bit of confidence." The appearance of the strands sets the scene and the tone for the whole assessment, as demonstrated in Table 1. In the assessment of Mrs. B, only one strand, *time,* is identified (see Table 2) and does not contribute greatly to a comprehensively coherent assessment. Its significance appears to simply fade away. It is initially raised by N2 in line 22 (Example 5) when she asks, "and how long have you been at this address." It recurs throughout the discourse but is never linked with the future, referring mainly to the present, the here and now. The past is referred to by N2 only when asking questions that refer to specific events (line 33).

Example 5

21	N2:	yes that's 63 J street (3) H town and how
22		long have you been here at this address
30	Mrs. B:	well I think that I've been here (3) I think I
31		came in June and I (1) it's either four or five

TABLE 1

The Introduction of Three Strands and Two Topics Within the
First Four Exchanges in the Assessment of Mrs. C by N1

Topic	Speaker	Text	Strand
Introductory	N1	Thank you for taking part in this research today	
		We're just going to be talking about you (3) and how you manage at home that sort of thing	
Nursing care		*We've been coming to you for #some months now haven't we	Time (1)
	Mrs. C	Yes	
Hygiene	N1	Helping you with your *showering you're starting to #feel better about that # now aren't you	Progress (Strand 3) Time (Strand 1)
	Mrs. C	Oh yes feeling more #confident too	Confidence (Strand 2)

Note. Mrs. C = patient; N1 = registered nurse.

TABLE 2

The Introduction of the Strand and One Topic Within the
First 17 Exchanges in the Assessment of Mrs. B by N2

Topic	Speaker	Text	Strand
Introductory indicating the frame	N2	And I'm going to *interview you if you don't mind on a few questions about yourself	
Demographic data	N2	(. . .) And #how long have you been at *this address	Time (1)

Note. Mrs. B = patient; N2 = nursing assistant.

```
32              years ago I forget now which
33   N2:        ⌐four or five⌐ years well we'll put four and
34   Mrs. B:    ⌐four or five⌐
35   N2:        a half about that that's fair
36   Mrs. B:    that'd be right yes
37   N2:        now your former occupation what were=
38   Mrs. B:    =well
39              of course I was a pensioner for some years
40   N2:        yes but prior to that
```

In sum we can say that a strand develops from a topic that does not
necessarily occur as a topic item on the assessment proforma but is one
that may be raised spontaneously in the conversation, often in different

contexts. A strand then recurs throughout the assessment and becomes effectively a recurring theme. Either speaker may address these themes from
different perspectives. They return to the assessment topic items already
addressed but from different perspectives, giving them a different focus—
for example, a statement is made that integrates *mobility* into everyday living and also into other topics. Such a strategy makes assessment meaningful for Mrs. C because topics so addressed are associated with her reality.
This point is demonstrated in the following extracts (Examples 6 and 7):

Example 6

124	N1:	yeah you look nice and strong on your legs
125		it's a while since you've been out isn't it
126	Mrs. C:	yeah I haven't been out what do you mean
127		out of the house
128	N1:	outside yeah
129	Mrs. C:	I haven't been out at all
130		no but you're going to want to get out aren't you
131	Mrs. C:	yeah
132	N1:	we talked about that extended day care but you
133		didn't seem interested in that are you not
134	Mrs. C:	no no I've got too many friends that I can't
135		keep up with them
136	N1:	yeah and they pop in and you play a good game
137		of cards I hear don't you

Example 7

379	Mrs. C:	now I haven't been to see the butcher
380		since March he'll wonder where I am unless as
381		somebody I don't know and the lady who has shop
382	N1:	it's only close isn't it but you've got that little hill
383	Mrs. C:	yes and I think I'll take the stick out
384	N1:	oh I would
385	Mrs. C:	I've got that stick
386	N1:	don't venture out without that stick
387	Mrs. C:	I've got that stick until July
388	N1:	that's right you've had it on loan from the
389		hospital what we'll do=

In each of these examples we can identify how the topic of *mobility* (appearing as an item on the proforma) is associated with other assessment items. Earlier in Example 4 (line 14), *mobility* is associated with *safety* and *hygiene* ("there's a nice support in that shower with the rail"). Later, in Example 6 (line 134), it is also linked with *social activities* ("friends") and attendance at "day care." In Example 7 (lines 379–386) it is associated with activities of daily living (shopping). It would appear that the achievement of a comprehensively coherent text demands that the discourse be coconstructed by both participants. The coherence generated in the discourse of N1 and Mrs. C is in part achieved by both nurse and patient redirecting the topic by changing its focus, the topics being signaled by lexical items (which thus become markers and will now be referred to as *lexical markers*).

Lexical markers need to be defined because the categories within which some have been placed in Table 3 may be difficult to justify. The participants appear to have made links between items that might be understood only by themselves and others who have in-depth knowledge of their particular situation (e.g., the "loan" of the stick from the hospital). Although the lexical items are not formally related semantically, there is nonetheless a meaning relationship (in the domain of nursing and the subdomain of assessment) that is not adventitious, and one in which members of the discourse community both recognize and orient to (Swales, 1990). In short, items may be semantically quite unrelated to other lexical markers of a topic and, in that they trigger a connection in the minds of one or both participants, there is, in that sense, a semantic relation. The interlocutors are enabled to engage in an uninterrupted flow of conversation. The storyline track is maintained, and the voice of the life world (cf. Mishler, 1984) is accommodated to move the interaction along. These triggers and markers allow the participants to discuss topics comprehensively and in depth. In the search for comprehensive coherence these links

TABLE 3
Examples of Topics and Their Lexical Markers in the Assessment of Mrs. C by N1

Topics	Lexical Markers of Coherence
Age	Eighty, eighty three, eighty four, looks terrific
Diet	Meals-on-wheels, sweets, meals, soups, fish mornay, supplies
Hospitalization	Diarrhea, diabetes, blood pressure, hospital visits
Hygiene	Showering, rail, skin, bath mat, washer
Investigations	Results, blood, glucose (levels)
Mobility	Stick, going out, strong on your legs, back steps, sister, walk

Note. Mrs. C = patient; N1 = registered nurse.

are vital, often providing a bridge between one topic and another. In this way *mobility* is at once firmly connected later in the assessment with "sister," on whom Mrs. C relies for physical support when visiting the hairdresser. Similarly, "looks terrific" is a marker of *age* because it refers directly to Mrs. C's chronological age. N1 can confidently assume that Mrs. C understands these connections, and without taking up unnecessary conversational space the interlocutors are able to move the interaction along rapidly and coherently. The relation between lexical items and a topic is not, however, simply a matter of semantics; it is also one of institutional and, in this case, professional meanings. There is a special connotation in a particular context. Lexical markers sometimes occur under more than one topic heading, for example "rail" occurs as a lexical marker of *hygiene* and also of *safety* (Example 4, lines 13–14). This repetition is demonstrated in Example 8 when it is seen that "husband" (line 29) is the lexical marker that signals the topic of *marriage* and *widowhood* (line 31) and later is linked to the markers of *socioeconomic status* (lines 42–50).

Example 8: N1 and Mrs. C

29 Mrs. C: my husband would walk through the house and put
30   on every light in every room but that's men you know
31 N1:   how long have you been widowed
32 Mrs. C: er last Christmas fifteen years
. . .
41 Mrs. C: yes
42 N1:   er you were saying the other day that you retired
43   here and took over a little business when you retired
. . .
49 N1:   what sort of work did you and your husband do before that
50 Mrs. C: clerical
51 N1:   both of you
52 Mrs. C: yeah

The discussion of the topics raised in the discourse of N1 and Mrs. C is exemplified in Table 3. The topics are related to a number of lexical markers that facilitate topic coherence. There are, for example, 16 lexical markers associated with *normalcy* (not shown), 7 associated with *diet,* 6 with *mobility,* and lexical markers of other topics ranging in number from 2 to 12. In an informal conversation, lexical markers function to indicate the topics and by reusing the item, topic areas may be broadened. When the text is

TABLE 4
The Reintroduction of Topics by Each Participant

Topic	Times Introduced by N1	Times Reintroduced by Mrs. C
Mobility	2	3
Nursing care	1	3
Hospitalization	0	1
Hygiene	1	3
Safety	0	1
Normalcy	4	1
Diet	0	1
Health status	0	1
Time management	0	1
Health care	1	1
Social support	1	9

Note. N1 = registered nurse; Mrs. C = patient.

analyzed for the reintroduction of topics, Mrs. C reintroduces topics throughout the text on 25 occasions and N1 on 10 (see Table 4). Topics that are reintroduced are those that are salient to the person introducing them, or to the activity, namely the assessment, or both. It can be seen that some topics such as *mobility* are raised and then expanded a number of times; others such as *hearing, dental health,* and *skin care* are raised only once. A topic that N1 identified as significant for Mrs. C was that of *social support.* Mrs. C was allowed the floor and reintroduced it nine times. By strategically responding to Mrs. C, N1 was able to coconstruct the assessment with her. Such situations support the view of Faulkner (1992) that, given the opportunity, the patient will volunteer information that is perceived to be significant. It is information that would not of necessity have been elicited in the strict question–answer sequences seen in the assessment of Mrs. B by N2.

COHERENCE AND THE ACHIEVEMENT OF DISCOURSAL GOALS

Topic Control and the Activation of Ideas

Although it is interesting to identify who it is who generally controls the topic exchange, because such control reflects the power relations in the interaction, it is also appropriate to determine the conditions under which the discourse of a rich and in-depth assessment can be coherently constructed. In relation to the discourse of N1 and Mrs. C, Button and Casey's (1984) work on the use of topic-initial elicitors is valuable. They proposed that the features of such elicitors can be summarized as follows: (a) topic-initial elicitors segment talk; (b) though making news inquiries they do not, themselves, present a newsworthy event; and (c) they provide an open, though bounded, domain from which events may be selected and offered as possible topic initials (Button & Casey, 1984, p. 171). Example 9 exemplifies and supports their argument.

Example 9: N1 and Mrs. C

```
07  N1:      helping with your showering you're starting to
08           feel better about that now aren't you
09  Mrs. C:  oh yes feeling more confident too
10  N1:      mm that's good
11  Mrs. C:  but as I say you know if I didn't feel well and I was (   )
12           I wouldn't have=
```

Line 10, for instance, indicates the termination of the segment begun in line 7. It does not present a newsworthy event in itself but it did, however, allow a further elicitation of topics in line 11 and 12. Such analysis as this provides the means for useful explanation for "local coherence." However, to pursue the notion of coherence at a deeper psychological level, we need to determine the cognitive functioning of participants in the interaction that allows topics to be reintroduced, sometimes much later in the interaction. Here, Chafe (1992) offered a useful perspective when he argued for ideas in discourse being in an "active" or "semiactive" state. In essence he proposed that there is a limit to a person's cognitive capacity, and sooner or later "active" ideas—that is, topics within the discourse—must lose their active status, making room for new ideas. He argued that ideas do not immediately become inactive when not being talked about but enter a state of "semiactivity" from which they can be subsequently triggered into the "active" state.

The discourse of Mrs. C and N1 provides useful evidence for Chafe's (1992) proposal. It demonstrates by the initiating and revisiting of topics that a large number of topic areas are in this semiactive state and are thus in an accessible "holding pattern." They are retrieved at different points during the assessment, with the strands *time, confidence,* and *progress* being accessed on numerous occasions. Topics are raised, dealt with immediately—sometimes in only one or two utterances—and then become inactive, not raised again in the interaction. These topics become part of the nursing history of Mrs. C, a pool of knowledge to be reactivated as necessary in future assessment and care. Much of this is recorded by the nurse and so becomes not only an event that is shared by N1 and Mrs. C, and thus part of their member resources, but a body of knowledge available to *any* nurse who continues with Mrs. C's care. In these instances, the topics never completely decay but are retained in written mode in nursing notes that constitute the completed assessment proforma. On occasions when a topic is not recorded or raised again, it is reasonable to believe that it can remain in the conversational consciousness of the participants to be made use of and referred to at a later date. (This, of course, assumes continuity of care by the same nurse—the ideal but not always the reality.) Eventually, however, a topic must decay with the degree of memory decay of the participants and thus become inaccessible.

EXTENDING THEORY: TRIGGERING FACTORS IN THE ACTIVATION AND REACTIVATION OF IDEAS

The ability to construct a coherent discourse is a general competence that one cannot necessarily assume, even less so in the context of assessment given that the topics are many and varied. Establishing comprehensive coherence involves making links between propositions and between sentences and sequences of sentences, and establishing these links within the overall framework of the activity. Assessment is also about connectedness; it is about the impact of one element on another. The social nature of an individual is not just about one area of that person's existence (e.g., the closeness of the daily network), but about how that network affects the person's physical state, care, functioning, and well-being, and the consequent emotional security of the person—and the family unit.

Central to Chafe's (1992) argument is the crucial presence of triggers, which we represent by the lexical indicators discussed earlier and by the strands that run through the discourse.

CONCLUSION

By examining in detail the interaction of one nurse–patient dyad (N1 and Mrs. C) and contrasting it with the interaction between a second dyad (N2 and Mrs. B), I propose conditions for the conduct of comprehensively coherent and therapeutic discourse. Comprehensive coherence is established by developing strands that serve as attentional tracks to maintain the assessment within the informal conversation frame and the nursing activity. Further, in this article I present arguments for an extension of Chafe's (1992) theory, proposing that semiactive ideas are activated by identifiable links in the form of lexical triggers that allow earlier topics to be reactivated and be present so that comprehensively coherent discourse can be achieved.

In this article, I analyzed and discussed the discourse of a nurse who does not take risks and compared it with that of the nurse with greater member resources who takes risks—in the framing of the activity and in the topic management—so that comprehensively coherent discourse, rich in assessment data, can be produced. The nurse, who can be identified as an expert, achieves this comprehensive coherence by coauthoring the discourse of a professional activity with the patient:

> The expert performer no longer relies on an analytic principle (rule, guideline, maxim) to connect her or his understanding of the situation to an appropriate action. The expert nurse, with an enormous background of experience, now has as intuitive grasp of each situation and zeroes in on the accurate region of the problem without wasteful consideration of a large range of unfruitful alternative diagnoses and solutions. (Benner, 1984, pp. 31–32)

REFERENCES

Benner, P. (1984). *From novice to expert: Excellence and power in clinical nursing practice.* Menlo Park, CA: Addison-Wesley.

Bourdieu, P. (1991). *Language and symbolic power.* Cambridge, England: Polity.

Bourdieu, P. (1993). *The field of cultural production.* Cambridge, England: Polity.

Briggs, C. L. (1986). *Learning how to ask: A sociolinguistic appraisal of the role of the interview in social science research.* Cambridge, England: Cambridge University Press.

Buber, M. (1966). In M. Friedman (Ed.), *The knowledge of man: A philosophy of the interhuman* (R. G. Smith, Trans.). New York: Harper & Row.

Button, G., & Casey, N. (1984). Generating topic: The use of topic initial elicitors. In J. M. Atkinson & J. Heritage (Eds.), *Structures of social action* (pp. 160–190). Cambridge, England: Cambridge University Press.

Candlin, S. (1997). *Towards excellence in nursing: An analysis of the discourse of nurses and patients in the context of health assessments.* Unpublished doctoral dissertation, Lancaster University, Lancaster, England.

Chafe, W. (1992). The flow of ideas in a simple written language. In W. C. Mann & S. A. Thompson (Eds.), *Discourse description: Diverse linguistic analyses of a fundraising text* (pp. 267–294). Amsterdam: Benjamins.

Fairclough, N. (1989). *Language and power.* London: Longman.

Faulkner, A. (1992). *Effective interaction with patients.* Edinburgh, Scotland: Churchill Livingstone.

Garfinkel, H. (1967). *Studies in ethnomethodology.* Englewood Cliffs, NJ: Prentice-Hall.

Goffman, E. (1967). *Interaction ritual: Essays on face-to-face behavior.* New York: Anchor.

Goffman, E. (1974). *Frame analysis.* New York: Harper & Row.

Jefferson, G. (1984). On stepwise transition from talk about a trouble to inappropriately next-positioned matters. In J. M. Atkinson & J. Heritage (Eds.), *Structures of social action* (pp. 191–222). Cambridge, England: Cambridge University Press.

Jones, R. (1996). *Responses to AIDS awareness discourse: A cross-cultural frame analysis* (Research Monographs No. 10). Hong Kong: City University of Hong Kong.

Mishler, E. (1984). *The discourse of medicine: Dialects of medical interviews.* Norwood, NJ: Ablex.

Morrison, P. (1994). *Understanding patients.* London: Baillière Tindall.

Riberio, B. T. (1996). Conflict talk in a psychiatric discharge interview: Struggling between personal and official footings. In C. R. Caldas-Coulthard & M. Coulthard (Eds.), *Texts and practices: Readings in critical discourse analysis* (pp. 179–193). London: Routledge.

Rogers, C. R. (1967). *On becoming a person: A therapist's view of psychotherapy.* London: Constable.

Swales, J. (1990). *Genre analysis: English for academic and research settings.* Cambridge, England: Cambridge University Press.

Research on Language and Social Interaction, 35(2), 195–218
Copyright © 2002, Lawrence Erlbaum Associates, Inc.

Expert Talk in Medical Contexts:
Explicit and Implicit Orientation to Risks

Per Linell
Viveka Adelswärd
Lisbeth Sachs
Margareta Bredmar
Department of Communication Studies
Linköping University

Ulla Lindstedt
University College of Health Sciences
Jönköping University

In medical contexts, parties often have reasons to focus on risks: risks of developing diseases or of having children with congenital diseases, risks involved in taking drugs or in using a particular type of therapy, and so forth. In such risk-implicative contexts, doctors and nurses deal with the risk topics sometimes directly, at other times quite indirectly. In this article, we discuss results from studying 5 different health care contexts. We discuss contextual factors that might account for some of the considerable differences in risk talk. Our claim is that the different explicit ver-

Work on this article was supported by research grants B91:0058 from the Swedish Council for Social Research to Per Linell, The Bank of Sweden Tercentenary Foundation 1995-5123 to Per Linell, and the Swedish Cancer Society (Cancerfonden, Grant Nos. 932658, 963605) to Lisbeth Sachs.

This article was presented at the I.A.D.A. Conference, Birmingham, April 9, 1999. An earlier version was read at a workshop on Institutional Discourse, 19 Nordiske Sociologikongress, København, June 14, 1997.

We wish to thank Sally and Chris Candlin, Srikant Sarangi and Roger Säljö for valuable comments on earlier drafts of this article.

Correspondence concerning this article should be sent Per Linell, Department of Communication Studies, Linköping University, SE-581 83   Linköping, Sweden.

sus implicit orientations are linked to where and how the different health care experts position themselves vis-à-vis scientific risk formulations and everyday risk perceptions. Our data on the implicit orientations to risk cast doubt on theories of discourse that would hold that all relevant understandings in discourse are made verbally manifest.

In this article, we deal with a specific aspect of expert talk, namely health care professionals (doctors, nurses, midwives) talking about risks: risks of contracting diseases, risks of having a disabled baby, and risks involved in specific types of medication or medical treatments. Drawing on data from varied health care contexts, we explore different modes of risk discourse. There appear to be quite distinct ways in which the expert role in the specific activity type encourages the incumbent to orient explicitly or implicitly either to scientific risk formulation or to everyday risk perception.

Risk is a negatively loaded concept. As a first approximation, we may say that it means (considerable) probability that something develops in an unfortunate or undesirable way, or that some negative event will occur in the future: *Collins English Dictionary* (1991) says "the possibility of incurring misfortune or loss; hazard" (p. 1336).

Calculation of risk is a typical feature of late modern society (Beck, 1992; Douglas, 1992; Giddens, 1991; Lupton, 1993). The meaning, measuring, and communication of risk have changed, for example, with more sophisticated statistics and computer facilities. Furthermore, with advanced medical technology more anomalies in the human body can be detected, and hence more people appear to be at risk. Not surprisingly, considerable research is currently being undertaken in different disciplines relating to risk, for example, medical risk, risk behavior, risk discourse, and the concept of risk itself. We do not address all of these fields, nor do we further dwell on issues of definition. Instead, we briefly introduce three points concerning the concept of risk in relation to health care discourse.

First, there are important differences between practitioners of science (e.g., medicine) and people in the everyday mundane world with regard to how they talk about risk. In science, a *risk* is a mathematically expressed probability that is defined and rendered meaningful only at the aggregational level of a population. A risk is expressed as the statistical likelihood of the occurrence of an event. Regarding individuals, risks are often deduced from a combination of such knowledge of statistical distribution in populations and the individuals' test results in the form of numerical values. These forms of expressing risks may differ in several respects, but they both concern objective, anonymized knowledge. In the everyday world, and for the individual human being, on the other hand *risk* means anxiety about the future, fear, or danger, that is, something emotionally highly charged that is threatening on a personal level: threats to one's welfare, well-being, health, maybe life. In this perspective, risk is a lived dimension of life, and "[h]igh risk means a lot of danger" (Douglas, 1992, p. 3).

Second, the previously mentioned point has an important corollary in clinical practice. Although health care professionals can talk about risk in scientific terms among themselves, they must, in their clinical practices, "recontextualize" (Linell, 1998) something that is meaningful only at the statistical level of probability within a population in such a way that it applies to the individual patient (Adelswärd & Sachs, 1998). This is a situation typical of modern predictive and preventive health care—which is concerned with the possibility of making scientifically objective statements about health risks—and at the same time it addresses individual human beings. The individual might be interested in the level of risk he or she is subject to, but usually the relevant issue is more of an all-or-nothing than some kind of a percentage issue; the individual might ask, "Am I, or will I get sick or not?" At the same time, some medical risks are subject to scientific controversy; there may be a range of professional uncertainty as to whether a certain value, say a high cholesterol value, constitutes a true risk factor. Balancing uncertainties in risk talk is difficult.

Third, in the domain of medical science, risk is part of cognitive understanding. It is not a bodily state or process (but interestingly, it is sometimes talked about as if it were; see Adelswärd & Sachs, 1998). There may be no obvious signs of deviance in one's body or one's environment that one can sense directly. However, once a person knows that she or he is at risk, the person often starts to feel uneasy; it is possible that she or he begins to feel sick and indeed becomes sick. Talk about diseases, diagnoses, and also risks may cause anxiety, psychosomatic symptoms, and the subjective experiences of illness. Risk discourse, it appears, is itself risky (Adelswärd & Sachs, 1998).

Therefore, talking to patients about risks is a delicate matter. Risk talk may seem necessary for patients to get the kind of knowledge that might motivate them to take measures, such as those of undergoing a certain medical treatment or changing their lifestyle. On the other hand, informing patients about risks may induce anxiety and indeed illness. Topics such as certain lifestyle issues are also threatening to personal integrity and therefore interactionally sensitive (Adelswärd & Sachs, 1996; Linell & Bredmar, 1996). Therefore, risk talk must combine knowledge claims with emotional dimensions.

If we consider medical professionals such as doctors and nurses as experts, risk talk is part of their "expert talk." Such talk involves both professional and institutional aspects (Sarangi & Roberts, 1999). Professionals are experts on measuring and assessing risks, and they can do so using biomedical (scientific) formulations. However, professionals are also part of institutional structures, and they differ in their proximity or distance to such expertise: Who can measure it? Who has access to the full significance of it? Who can only communicate? Who is authorized to convey information? Informing about risk in a professional manner and in institutional contexts is far from a straightforward matter. One may have to make compromises between scientific formulations and everyday perceptions, between biomedical considerations and emotional and moral dimensions, and between expert knowledge and institutional constraints. There may be contexts in which health professionals choose to engage in information giving rather explicitly and other contexts in which they prefer to express themselves in implicit ways, or even to remain silent about the risks involved. Our aim in this article was to compare risk discourse from five different health care sites in which at least one of the parties clearly orients to risk(s) in the interaction. The five different situations were selected to provide for a sociopragmatic variation regarding how risk talk is handled. This variation is obviously attributable to a host of factors, and the purpose of this study was to identify some such factors.

DATA

We refer to five different corpora of Swedish health care discourse that are derived from the following sites:

1. Genetic information talks ($n = 33$), where a specialist in genetics talks to a person who suspects that she or he is at high risk of developing cancer because of hereditary factors (Adelswärd & Sachs, 1998).
2. Health information talks ($n = 28$), where a nurse talks with a male client who has, or has had, or may develop, high cholesterol values (Adelswärd & Sachs, 1996).

3. Booking interviews in maternal health care ($n = 43$), where a mid-wife talks with a pregnant woman (in about the 10th week of pregnancy) about a test (alpha-feto-protein or AFP) to be administered later (Week 16), which (if the woman chooses to take it) can indicate fetal anomalies[1] (Linell & Bredmar, 1996).

4. Medical testing situations ($n = 44$), routine medical checkups that are regular parts of midwife and pregnant woman encounters (data were collected in the same project as Site 3). These encounters take place later in pregnancy than the booking interview. Here, we are concerned with the episodes in which physical or physiological measurements and test results are reported and assessed (Bredmar, 1999; Bredmar & Linell, 1999).

5. Talk during urography and kidney radiography ($n = 10$), where a nurse and a patient talk during a kidney X-ray examination; we focus here on talk before and during the nurse's administering of an intravenous (and potentially risky) injection of contrast fluid (Lindstedt, 1997).

In the following, we discuss these five health care situations with regard to how parties orient to relevant risks. Space restrictions force us to use only one or two excerpts for each site, but we have chosen examples that are quite typical of the respective situations.

ANALYSIS

The genetic information talks are part of a consultation service for the genetic assessment of risk of developing cancer. Clients have contacted specialists at a university hospital to find out more about their risk status. The data used here concern women who so far are quite healthy but suspect that they may develop breast (or ovarian) cancer because they have had several close relatives with the disease. The talks were based on genealogical mapping and information about the family's disease history, with no data from blood DNA tests.[2] In the corpus of genetic information talks, doctors always talk explicitly and at length about risks:[3]

(1) (GI: Dr. A, Pt. 29: 150–154) (D = doctor, P = patient)

1 D: (. . .) but then there are those who are not
2   prepared to run any risk at all and they, so

3		you, those who have been operated in Sweden
4		they have had roughly, they have been in
5		families that have had a 50 percent risk of
6		being genetic carriers, maybe then a 40
7		percent risk of disease, approximately. but
8		then there are also those who have run about
9		half that risk, around 25 percent that is, who
10		have been, if you say that this, if this had
11		been a family with a lot of sick members and
12		so to say then children of a sick person run a
13		50 percent risk, while a man, here one doesn't
14		really know, he will not get sick ((*D is*
15		*pointing to the genogram*))
16	P:	no--
17	D:	yes that's right, so the girls here so to say,
18		the grandchildren of, if there was a person
19		with the disposition here, ((*pointing to*
20		*genogram*)) only run half, that is 25 percent
21		risk of being, and there are those who have
22		chosen an operation also coz they find that
23		the risk has been unreasonable for them to
24		run, so that so that you feel yourself so to
25		say
26	P:	and as you thought then I should, so to say,
27		count it in percentages that it should be 20
28		percent or something for me
29	D:	yes, that's right. if you have a close
30		relative then at least a double risk, at least
31		20 percent risk then

As we can see, this short episode is replete with mention of "risk," the doctor using the word nine times, almost always in combination with a quantitative specification in "percent."[4] Apart from being related to substantially high risks, the explicit orientation to risk could have to do with the fact that we are faced with an expert authorized to comment on it. (In the following excerpts, we see several cases of nurses orienting less explicitly to risks.) The doctor in Excerpt 1 displays her expert knowledge in discussing, particularly in turn 1, risk calculation at a population level; it is a display of expert knowledge. Yet, all this information is addressed to a particular patient, and it is understood within this framing. There is also a certain ambiguity in the doctor's account between generalization and personalization and a tendency to slide from the former more into the latter as the talk proceeds. Some of the discursive strategies are anonymizing, that is, talk about other people ("those who are not prepared . . . ," "they have been in families . . .") and hypothetical case formulations ("if there was a person . . ."). The doctor's references are as a rule generalized to persons with certain given family incidences, but at the same time, they are tied to particular persons in the patient's genogram. The patient, for her part, concludes that her own risk is "20 percent or something," which is confirmed by the doctor ("at least 20 percent risk then"). When risks get talked about in individualized terms, they tend to become concretized, almost reified as if they were something "carried" by the patient in her own body. This effect is also produced by the clinicians' use of compounds such as "risk-organ, risk-person, high-risk-person, risk-family, risk-distance, risk-zone," and so forth (for more data, see Adelswärd & Sachs, 1998).

In the health information talks (site 2 previously), the patients are middle-age, apparently healthy men without any symptoms of disease. They have been offered a health checkup within a special preventive survey program within a primary health care setting, with respect to risk factors for cardiovascular disease and particularly risks of incurring coronary heart disease. Data come from the nurse's talk with the men about their health status as indicated by test values:

(2) (HI: A2) (The nurse [N] is referring to test values recorded in the client's [C] file.)

```
1    N:   (. . .) the cholesterol is due to the fat things
2         and triglycerides to all the sweet things. the
3         cholesterol, here you have 8.0 ((points to
4         table of figures)) and there one has a limit
5         of 6.8 so you are in fact a little bit above
6         so one has to look a bit here at what you eat-
7    C:   I see, here it is the food of course--
8    N:   it doesn't have to be, there might of course
9         be a small hereditary part also
     ((7 turns omitted))
10   N:   but it is of course the diet very much then--
11        take a look at the milk here, you drink
12        real milk, and the butter and, well, there
13        are many things one can take a look at, one
```

14	will have to go into the diet there and then
15	one has the hereditary factor too to look
16	at--. so you lie here, at 8.0 and 6.8 one
17	should be at at most then, that is the limit
18	one has taken--. and then we have the
19	triglycerides, all the sweet things, and you
20	lie at 2.4, 2.4 and 2.5 is what one may have
21	there so you lie exactly at the limit so
22	that's why I've written this in red you see--
23	((*points to figures in red ink*)). so that
24	there you have all the sweet things, coffee
25	cakes, biscuits--, juice--

The numerical exactness in this piece of health information talk ("6.8," "8.0," etc.) gives it a flavor of scientific expert talk and its associated authority (Adelswärd & Sacks, 1998). Expert talk is accomplished in explaining what is normal or average, the norms referring to charts derived from studies of populations. Yet, we have here too a situation in which the individual case must be addressed and accommodated to general knowledge. We find extensive talk about lifestyle issues, for example, about diet such as drinking milk and eating sweet cakes (lines 11–12, 19, 24–25, etc.); such issues have become culturally assumed to be (partly) the patient's responsibility. Therefore, they are also potentially face threatening.

In the health information talks, there are relatively few explicit mentions of the word *risk,* but the talk about numerical test values and numerical "limits" implicates a perspective of risk. In a few talks ($n = 8/30$), the word *risk* is in fact used but not with such exact measures as in the genetic information talks mentioned earlier. Here are a few short excerpts:

(3a) (HI: M2)

1	N:	you have been a smoker since you were fourteen
2		years old, but you know about the risks, there
3		are a lot of dangerous poisons one inhales,
4		consciously you know.

(3b) (HI: F2)

| 1 | N: | it is this fitness-keeping part and tobacco, |
| 2 | | alcohol, diet and exercise that one takes a |

3	look at specifically and the age of forty and
4	one--, it's these risk factors one has that one
5	ought to peep at a bit and it is good of course
6	if one is aware of it oneself and can draw the
7	boundaries, you know, that one keeps within the
8	normal. then it was the exercise and there at
9	least once a week trying hard, what do you do?

Note that the nurse in (3b) characteristically uses the term *risk factor*, thus arguably distancing herself a bit from the face-threatening topic of risks. Moreover, many of the nurse's statements in the health information talks are made in a general, anonymizing form, using "one" (Swedish *man*) or "you" (Swedish *du*), the latter often ambiguous between the generic and the personal interpretations. The nurse talks in general terms rather than delivering individual diagnoses, and she is primarily focused on interpreting the measurement values: that is, she orients to the task as a medical expert engaged in information giving. Her advice giving is rendered ambiguous partly along the lines described by Silverman (1997) in his study of discourses of counselling.[5] Yet she asks about the patient's habit ([3b] line 9: "what do you do?"; i.e., in terms of physical exercise) or points to risky habits ([3a] line 1: "you have been a smoker . . ."). However, she is quite cautious not to issue explicit warnings or advice, except when a high cholesterol value is combined with a high glucose tolerance value (not shown here). She is evidently doing elaborate face work in coping with sensitive topics, especially with regard to drinking habits (Adelswärd & Sachs, 1996).

In the case of the booking interviews with the expectant mothers, the clients are all healthy, and there is no reason to assume (at least not at this stage of pregnancy) that they are subject to heightened individual risks. However, the topic of the optional AFP test is always taken up by the midwife, and in some of the encounters (particularly with first-time mothers) there is explicit talk about fetal anomalies. The implicit message is of course that any pregnancy runs a (small) risk of developing in such a way. Often, the physical and physiological conditions are described in an information-giving mode (cf. Sarangi & Clarke, 2002), as in (4):

(4) (Tema K: BU1) (Excerpt from episode on AFP test; M = midwife,
    W = pregnant woman [first pregnancy])

1	M:	and this blood test, it shows then that if one
2		has heightened values of (.) °alpha-feto-

```
 3        proteins, that is a protein which is found in
 4        the blood.° and that can, has one got too much
 5        of it, that can indicate that there's
 6        something (0.5) which is not well with the
 7        baby, °you see°
 8   W:   °mm-hm°
 9   M:   an' (.) what one can see then above all, it's
10        those (.) open (.) spinal hernias
11   W:   mm. °mm°
12   M:   one can also then, often in combination with
13        those it can be that they don't have (.) that
14        much brain either
15   W:   °°I see°°
16   M:   plus abdominal (2.5) ah hernia, that (1.5) the
17        abdominal wall is not closed so to speak, you
18        see
19   W:   °mm°
20   M:   but the bowels °so to speak get out like
21        this°. and-ah (.) it is of course not that (.)
22        *dangerous* after all, you see, but it's just
23        that it's good to know about it.
24   W:   °.yes°
25   M:   .hh ah well, so there you have an option to
26        take such a test.
27   W:   mm.
28   M:   now I should also tell you that this is of
29        course very uncommon, both these things.
30   W:   it is, yes.
31   M:   yes, it is, so that it is so to speak
32        *nothing* which ⌈(.)
33   W:                  ⌊no
34   M:   often happens, but it's terribly uncommon.
```

There is also talk (not shown in the excerpt) about the fact that the woman may end up in a situation in which she must make the difficult decision about whether to undergo an abortion or not. That is, we sometimes get a rather detailed description of frightful medical conditions, but there is no explicit use of the term *risk*. There is also a frequent striving to avoid going into concrete matters when it can be avoided (see Linell & Bredmar, 1996).

Moving on to the medical testing situations (with partly the same women as in the booking interviews), in our article (see Bredmar & Linell, 1999, for more material) we only address what happens when the midwife has found deviant test results; that is, results that might indicate some threat to the pregnancy or to the child.

(5) (Tema K: B6:5:5) (W = first-time mother; M has just measured
    a somewhat deviant symphysis-fundus (S-F) measure[6])

```
 1   M:   <now what I'll do> (.) in fact here is that
 2        since you ended up below this (.) lower normal
 3        curve so to speak ⌜(0.2) then I put
 4   W:              ⌞ye:s
 5   M:   a minus there, an' it is bec- it only means
 6        that you are below the broken line, it's ⌜it's
 7   W:                          ⌞ye:s
 8   M:   so that if you wonder why what it is
 9   M:   I'm wri⌜ting
10   W:       ⌞ye:s
11   M:   and the head is quite clearly fixed, it is
12        terrifically (.) well (0.2) ⌜anchored
13   W:                 ⌞down
14        (0.2)
15   M:   m⌜m
16   W:   ⌞mm
17   M:   (0.2) .hh fetal sounds they counted here I see
18        an' they write W N, means without notice
19        ⌜(0.3) I won't count it but I'll—
20   W:   ⌞ye:s
```

M notes that the S-F value falls outside of the normal range (lines 5–6). However, rather than commenting on its significance, she just describes what kind of note she makes in the file ("I put a minus there"). She then goes on to mention some other things that are positive (lines 11, 17). Incidentally, notice that M starts this with "and" (line 11) when perhaps we could have expected "but." The use of "and" implies that the prior information was not really negative. Nevertheless, what M does is to arrange for W to come back for one or two extra checkups, which is definitely outside of normal routines (this cannot be seen in the excerpt). Therefore, the perception of risk results in certain kinds of institutional procedures outside of the discourse in a narrow sense.

In other cases, M would try to discursively neutralize unexpected deviations. In general, midwives seem to avoid mentioning alarming situations (nor are there any comments of the type "nothing to worry about"). They tend to ameliorate negative features, or at least they refrain from commenting on them. Risky aspects are mitigated or minimized in talk and never thematized in linguistic terms by the midwife; that is, she does not use the word *risk*. Similar findings have been reported by Leppänen (1998), who observed Swedish district nurses visiting patients in their homes.

Finally, the kidney X-ray examination (site 5) itself involves certain risks because a few patients may develop strong and rapid allergic reactions to the contrast fluid (risk of suffocation). The nurses ask questions about allergic dispositions that are motivated by the medical risks. That is, the risks motivate these discoursal ingredients—the questions—but at the same time, the topical aspect of risk is completely disguised; there is never any mention of risks, not even an implicit orientation to it. However, in contrast to the earlier example, we have here the perception of risk realized at the interactional level in another way. The nurses observe carefully the patients in the minutes after the injection, often filling the time with small talk. We just cite a few sequences illustrating these two kinds of episodes. Excerpt 6 occurs quite early in the encounter:

(6) (Tema K: UR7: 25–41) (The nurse has just asked if the patient has undergone an X-ray examination before.)

```
1   N:   it went well then, you didn't feel unwell from
2        it?
3   P:   no, though eh it was warm
4   N:   a little warm one will most often get from it.
5        (.) otherwise (.) you haven't got any allergy?
6   P:   no:
7   N:   diabetes?
8   P:   yes, asthma
9   N:   you have asthma?
10  P:   yes
```

```
11   N:   yes but it's nothing °current°
12   P:   but ah no, I don't think so
13   N:   but you can eat all kinds of food and such?
14   P:   ye:s
15   N:   diabetes?
16   P:   no
17   N:   you haven't got that either?
18   P:   no
19   N:   no. (.) °then let'see° ((proceeds to preparing
20        for the actual examination))
```

Here, the allergy question is smuggled in after some talk about previous X rays (line 5). The allergy and diabetes questions are always routinely asked, partly in a manner similar to (6), and there is never any motivation given by the nurse. Patients never ask for a reason for the question; although they might of course suspect that the reason is that the examination might cause allergic reactions, they are not informed about which aspect is crucial (the injection of the contrast fluid) or about the seriousness of the reaction, which can occur in exceptional cases. The talk occurring in connection with the actual injection never appears to make the topic of allergy relevant either. The injection episode from the same encounter as (6) is given in (7):

(7) (Tema K: UR7: 121 ff)

```
1    N:   then you know that you can get a little warm
2         from this contrast?
3    P:   mm
4    N:   this is of course not as much as you get when
5         you had your head X-ray- X-rayed ((N is here
6         referring to the amount of contrast fluid))
7    P:   no:=
8    N:   =barely half of it
9    P:   I see
10        ((45.0; the contrast fluid is being injected))
11   N:   °if we have got the time so we will follow the
12        time then°
13   P:   mm
14   N:   when one has got half of this contrast then §§
15        then we will start this watch an' then we take
```

```
16          after five minutes pictures of—
17   P:     .hja §§
18   N:     there is no odd feeling?
19   P:     °it's a bit warm in my arm°
20   N:     a little warm in your arm?
21   P:     mm
22          (8.0)
23   N:     but nothing tightening or anything?
24   P:     no it ⌈goes f-
25   N:          ⌊it didn't swell up I I shoot fairly
26          slowly
27   P:     it goes super
28   N:     mm
29          ((90.0))
```

As we can see, there is no mention on the part of the nurse of anything risky. Rather, she chooses to warn of a common feeling of warmth (lines 1–2), referring back to the previous X-ray the patient has had (lines 4–5). After the injection, she asks a neutral question, which the patient answers by referring precisely to the feeling of warmth (lines 18–19). This is followed by another question (line 23)—which does incorporate a more specific presupposition (about a possible feeling of "tightening")—but its negative formulation projects a preferred "no problems" response (cf. Heritage, 2000), and the patient aligns with the preference by simply confirming this (lines 24, 27). The same pattern is repeated in other encounters; (8) is another example:

(8) (Tema K: UR4: 104 ff) (N2 = assistant nurse)

```
 1   N:     so you'll get the contrast then
 2          (7.0)
 3   N:     °°here first a little here then°°
 4          (8.0)
 5   N:     now you can get a little warm (.) in your
 6          body (.) from this contrast
 7   P:     I see
 8   N:     but it (.) goes over directly when I
 9          finish shooting then
10   P:     mm I see
11   N:     if you feel something else you must tell
```

```
12         me
13    P:   yes °°but it's nothing°°
14         (18.0; more contrast fluid is being injected))
15    N2:  °well, then we start the watch°
16         (10.0)
17    N:   it feels well?
18    P:   yes it's noth-
19    N:   didn't feel anything?
20    P:   no:
21         (39.0)
```

The nurse repeats her neutral questions inquiring about any specific sensations at intervals (lines 11, 17, 19, and more times, not shown here, during the minutes that follow). The nurse attends to any signs of allergic reactions, but as the patient will be the first to sense anything, the nurse asks about it. Thus, her questions are clearly motivated by her awareness of risks, but they are all formulated in very neutral terms, avoiding any mention of *allergy* or *risk*. The frequency of the repeated questions ("how does it feel?") may communicate special concern, but the nurse balances this by the neutral formulation and by small talk in between (not shown here).

COMPARISON OF CONTEXTS

The different health care situations we have discussed involve quite divergent sorts of risk discourse. A few situations involve explicit discussions of risks, some carefully avoid all risk talk (although the knowledge of risks still motivates particular communicative acts, such as the questions in the nurses' urography talks), and some fall in between these extremes. A few describe possible "dreadful" futures (e.g., fetal anomalies in [4]), whereas most of them only hint at risks in the abstract. Why are these differences there? They may of course be due to such factors as personal habits and idiosyncratic strategies on the part of individual professionals and patients and the like. However, barring such factors (recall that we selected examples that are typical of the respective activity types), we can invoke the following features that distinguish the five situations.

1. First, is the *individual patient* already known (or assumed) to be (i.e., at the stage when the talks were recorded) *"at high risk"*—that is, at higher risk than an average person of the same age, sex, medical status, and so forth? This is clearly so in genetic information talks. Indeed, the patient herself often suspects it in these cases, even though there are also a few women who do not suspect that they are at high risk, but they still consult the specialist to get a confirmation that they are at low risk. In the other cases, the answer to the question posed is "no," except perhaps in health information talks where it may be "yes or no." Also in the medical testings (site 4), some women (those who have already shown deviant values?) may be regarded as "risk persons."

2. A second factor has to do with how close the risk is assumed to be in terms of a time perspective. Parties might be more inclined to talk about risks that may materialize within say 10 or 20 years (cf. genetic information, health information), whereas they refrain from talking about risks in cases in which the risks concern the near future (cf. the medical testings). This is also related to where the patient is in *relation to medical treatment*: Has a specific treatment been decided, or is it in fact already being administered? In the information-giving activity of the genetic information talks, parties are at a preparatory stage, but the patient may (have to) decide later whether to undergo medical treatment (e.g., surgical removal of the breasts). Following the information-oriented episodes of the maternal health care booking interviews, the women must likewise make a specific decision on a possible medical intervention; this (abortion) is potentially even more morally difficult because it directly involves another human being (the unborn child). At the same time, in these booking interviews—unlike the genetic information talks—the woman's pregnancy has already brought her under the medical surveillance of maternal health care. The health information talks (site 2) are less directly related to far-reaching interventions; these are information talks combined with health checkups, which are part of a general preventive health care program (rather than individually based). In the medical testing situations (site 4), the patient is under medical care, and there might seem to be no need to talk specifically about risks unless the patient wants to do so herself. Finally, in the urography situation, the patient is (in that very moment) undergoing a medical-technical examination that is preferably not interrupted or suspended there and then. It is a coercive situation with highly constrained choices.

3. The previous point is related to the third: What is the expected role of *"risk talk" within the whole talk activity* (encounter) as parties under-

stand it; that is, is talk about risks a point on the agenda of the encounter? In the genetic information talks, risk talk is indeed the point of the whole encounter; the clients are healthy persons who want to see the doctor precisely because they are already concerned about being at risk. This may account for the explicitness. Nonetheless, such talk can be staged in different ways, and we find a good deal of anonymizing strategies—that is, talk in general terms—on the part of the geneticist. In the health information context (site 2), the talk is oriented to matters of health rather than illness; in preventive health care, it is a question of how to preserve fitness. The clients are healthy persons who want to have their good health confirmed. Yet, the encounters take place against a horizon of risks; otherwise, there would have been no reason for a survey.

The point of the AFP test episode of the booking interviews is, arguably, also to bring up risks (i.e., those of having a child with physical anomalies). The midwife's talk often involves a detailed description of such anomalies, but the aspect of risk is often implicit, rather than made explicit, in such episodes. What midwives often do is to say that "such things are unusual," thus discursively trying to minimize risks. (However, "unusual" in this context may carry more weight than elsewhere.) The midwife seems to try to distance herself and her partner, the pregnant woman, from the dreadful risk by talking about anomalies in general terms, as something that can occur (in other persons?); she would never say, "You have an X percent risk of having a child with congenital defects." In addition, the AFP episode, which can sometimes be made very short, is just a small part of a much more comprehensive encounter oriented to normality in pregnancy and to inducing self-confidence (Bredmar & Linell, 1999). Although it clearly belongs to the midwives' official instructions to "assess risks" in the pregnancies they monitor, and risk assessments are indeed performed in their medical examinations, it appears that risks are strongly downplayed in talk (Bredmar, 1999). In our data, maternal health care encounters are quite simply not contexts for risk talk; that is, parties, and particularly midwives, strongly disprefer explicit talk about risks. In the case of the kidney X-ray examination, finally, the medical treatment has been deemed necessary on independent grounds and will be carried out, preferably without arousing the patient's alarm.

4. Related to this point are differences in the *professionals' responsibilities* and entitlements. There are status differences between doctors and nurses, for example, limits to nurses' rights to inform about diagnoses and the like.[7] Thus, the nurses in the situations presented here (sites 2–5) are

not ultimately responsible for all the information that can be given, whereas the geneticists in the genetic information talks are.

Responsibilities for information giving are related to the level and quality of professional knowledge and to issues of uncertainty (cf. S. Candlin, 2002). Specialists versus general practitioners, physicians versus nurses, and so forth have access to different kinds of information. In the field of genetic counseling, the knowledge bases have changed rapidly over time as a result of scientific discoveries. One may therefore assume that some aspects of risk talk in situations such as those we have discussed in this article (particularly perhaps in the case of genetic information giving and counseling) have changed, or will change, over a few years' time.

5. There is also a question of *time frames* (in another sense than the one mentioned previously in point 2). Professionals will allocate very different amounts of time to individual clients; for example, psychotherapists use plenty of time, whereas surgeons seem to give very little time. The genetic specialists in the genetic information talks spend considerable time with each client, whereas the midwives within maternal health care are involved in routinized encounters for which much less time has been assigned. The ongoing process of the X-ray examination in urography talks implies a particularly tight time constraint. Clearly, this influences which issues can be raised. In our cases, we may tentatively order the encounter types in terms of decreasing time frames: genetic information talks → health information talks → maternal health care booking interviews → maternal health care check-up visits → urography.

6. Regarding the *attribution* of risks *to different causes,* the situations are different. In the genetic information talks, parties deal with (heightened) risks that are thought to be due to genetic factors. The point of the AFP test raised in the maternal health care booking interview is to reveal fetal anomalies already present or to determine a heightened risk of developing fetal anomalies later. The women visiting the maternal health care center have come far into a natural process (i.e., pregnancy) that involves certain risks, but there is relatively little the individual woman can do about it. By contrast, cholesterol values (in the health information talks) are, it is argued, lifestyle related and therefore potentially self-inflicted. Finally, the urography situation is unique in that it is the medical examination itself that is inflicting certain risks. Yet, this treatment has been deemed necessary and is being carried out, despite these risks (unless, of course, there is evidence of hypersensitivity beforehand).

7. This brings us to a final point, that of *patient responsibility.* Can the patient influence the level of future risks, and if so, in what ways?

TABLE 1
Patient Responsibility

Variable	Source of Risks	Decision on Test or Treatment
1. Genetic information	No	Yes
2. Health information	Yes	Yes
3. AFP test	No	Yes
4. Routine medical test	No (Yes?)	No
5. Urography	No (Yes?)	No

Note. AFP = alpha-feto-protein.

Actually, there appear to be two aspects of this issue. First, are risks due to factors within the individual patient's control (see point 6)? Second, are patients co-responsible for deciding on further testings (production of further knowledge about risks), medical treatment, or both? The considerations on these points are summarized in Table 1.

Naturally, a table like this one needs a number of provisos. We have to ignore these in this context. One comment seems necessary, though, and this concerns the important question of *the impact of the talk itself.* Risk talk is not only a matter of talking about (preexisting) medical risks or conditions; one may take (or generate) risks depending on one's discoursal choices (S. Candlin, 2002). For example, it is often believed that if patients get stressed (i.e., if they are stressed by others or they stress themselves from getting to know about their own risks), this very attention to risks may influence the outcome. Stress is induced by knowledge of risk; it is a "medico-moral concept" (Harris, 1989). It is a matter of dispute whether this can affect the incidence of cardiovascular diseases (cf. the health information talks) or of cancer (cf. the genetic information talks). At any rate, the argument seems relevant for medical tests and measurements (site 4) and urography (which accounts for the affirmatives within parentheses in Table 1).

CONCLUSION: EXPLICIT AND
IMPLICIT RISK TALK

Professionals in medical settings relate to risk in different ways, for example, by explaining, discovering, controlling, and trying to eliminate it. In talk, they sometimes also ignore risk, at least on the surface. We have found a variation in risk talk, ranging from explicit talk about risks (including describing frightening scenarios and individualizing information), over implicit (or indirect) talk about risk (talk is risk implicative but not explicit about risk, and information tends to be anonymized), to clear avoidance of talk about risk. In the last-mentioned case, there are other nondiscursive kinds of orientation to risk; that is, the nurses (in the health information talks) and midwives (in the medical assessment situations of site 4) booking extra medical checkups (in cases of deviant values), or the nurses (in the urography situations) paying keen attention to signs of allergic reactions (also asking their neutral questions about it).

There is evidently a complex interaction of factors behind these differences. Our data are limited and do not warrant any definitive conclusions, but some hypotheses (to be further tested in future research) can be suggested. Explicitness is probable if (a) patients can, in and through their own conduct, influence future risks; (b) the individual patient is known to be at high risk; (c) the patient is in the process of being informed rather than being already under medical treatment; (d) the topic of risks is an agenda point rather than something that is more incidentally brought up; (e) the professional has the legitimized right to issue medical (predictive or diagnostic) information; and (f) there is plenty of time available. Implicitness or avoidance are chosen as professional strategies in cases where the opposite conditions are at hand. In addition, there are of course other factors, including the ideological difference between a traditional, paternalistic biomedical model and the philosophy of partnered care that implies informed decision making. Our hunch is that Swedish health care of the 1990s has been fairly geared to the latter, also in practice. The point is, however, that even if this is true, the complex interplay of factors will still necessarily generate a considerable amount of sociopragmatic variation in risk talk.

FINAL DISCUSSION

There are two kinds of issues that we raise as we approach the end. The first has to with how to interpret the notions of risk talk and expert talk, the latter being the common focus of the articles in this special issue. Both notions may be interpreted in different ways. *Risk talk* can mean both talking about risks (e.g., medical risks) and generating risks in talk; risk is constituted in and through particular discoursal choices (S. Candlin, 2002). We have dealt primarily with the first aspect, but we have also pointed to a possible, and intricate, interdependence between the two aspects.

As regards *expert talk,* one may understand this as talk exhibiting expertise; not all talk by experts is then indicative of expertise (or expert knowledge). In this article, we have treated expert talk simply as talk by professionals, whether it is marked in any special way or not. Admittedly, this is in one sense to trivialize the notion of expert talk. One may also, following Sarangi and Roberts (1999), want to distinguish between professional discourse and institutional discourse. The former would then refer to professionals' knowledge of their specialist domain and their skills to treat clients in a professional manner, whereas the latter would refer to the talk (and text) that is produced (mainly by professionals) as a consequence of both professional knowledge and various institutional constraints and empowerments. Nevertheless, we have included in our notion of expert talk not just the manifestation and use of professional (expert) knowledge but also of the institutional role of (being treated by self and other as) expert. As we have seen, medical professionals may have various reasons to display or censure their expert knowledge as they interact in different clinical contexts. Such reasons may have to do with the tension in orientation to both scientific formulations and everyday perceptions that is inherent in risk discourse (cf. the introduction). Therefore, although professional expertise obviously enters the picture, we argue that we are not yet in a position to identify exactly what features of discourse are expressive of expertise.

What we have done is to hint at a possible model of the relations between contextual factors and aspects of risk talk within health care systems. In doing so, we have not here analyzed patients' and clients' contributions to risk talk. However, our general observation is that risk talk, in the situations studied, is part of collaborative communicative projects led by, and typically initiated by, the professionals. The substantial part of the talk is actually produced by the latter. The predicament of many professionals can be discussed in terms of a communicative dilemma (Adelswärd, 1998): to give or not to give information, to talk about risks and possibly cause anxiety and worries or to avoid such talk and thereby perhaps prolong uncertainties and other kinds of worries. This also involves issues of face work. Many more studies of authentic risk talk are needed before we can formulate a more complete and descriptively adequate model. From there, we might then, with the help of other kinds of studies and in dialogue with medical professionals, start a discussion of normative import: What advice can be given to practitioners as to how to go about solving the dilemmas involved?

Our final point is a methodological one, which might be of some generality for discourse analysis, especially as far as institutional talk is concerned. There is a need for contextual, extraneous information in interpreting discourse data (cf. Cicourel, 1992; Hak, 1999). The analyst may be incapable of interpreting the discourse (at least as it is is intended by the professional) unless he or she has access to ethnographic information; that is, he or she knows about the professional background (e.g., medical motivation of allergy questions in the urography data). Yet, though we turn to such contextual dimensions in accounting for the way talk is organized and orchestrated, we are of course still doing *discourse* analysis, and it is in the discourse that we observe the "procedural consequentiality of context" (Peräkylä, 1997), that is, how contextual conditions are reflected in different kinds of risk discourse.

NOTES

1 Heightened values of AFP in the blood can indicate serious anomalies in the fetus.

2 At the time when this (first) data corpus was collected, it was not yet possible to analyze blood samples for detecting cancer genes. It is assumed that today 10% to 15% of breast cancer can be accounted for by means of this kind of gene technology.

3 The original data are Swedish, and our analyses reported here and elsewhere were of course carried out on the originals (which are available from the authors). Here, we present data in approximate English translations, and our discussion refers to points in the translated data. We follow the transcription conventions adopted within conversation analysis, but note the following deviations: * * surround talk with laughter in the voice, §§ denotes throat clearing, and -- marks an intonation designed to suggest that a continuation is possible but the speaker lets go of it.

4 Here, the physician tries to combine and quantify data of different origins and variable quality to present one final numerical estimation of risk. Many of the reasonings in the doctor's risk discourse appear to be, from a statistical point of view, highly questionable (Sachs, Taube, & Tishelman, 2001).

5 Silverman (1997) noted the following features, which he interpreted as devices for making utterances ambiguous between advice and information giving: "advice-as-information sequences" ("information-about-the-kind-of-advice-we-give-in-this-

clinic," p. 170), formulating hypothetical cases ("if so-and-so was the case, then . . ."), and using "oblique," often impersonal references to both the counseling agent ("we" rather than "I") and recipients ("one," "some people").

6 As a regular part of the expectant mother's visit to the maternal health care center, the midwife uses a measuring tape to measure the distance from the symphysis pubis to the top (fundus) of the uterus.

7 On legal constraints regarding the right to give advice in various situations (e.g., family planning and abortion), see C. Candlin and Lucas (1985).

REFERENCES

Adelswärd, V. (1998). Moral dilemmas and moral rhetoric in interviews with conscientious objectors. *Research on Language and Social Interaction, 31,* 439–464.

Adelswärd, V., & Sachs, L. (1996). A nurse in preventive work: Dilemmas of health information talks. *Scandinavian Journal of Caring Sciences, 10,* 45–52.

Adelswärd, V., & Sachs, L. (1998). Risk discourse: Recontextualization of numerical values in clinical practice. *Text, 18,* 191–210.

Beck, U. (1992). *Risk society.* London: Sage.

Bredmar, M. (1999). *Att göra det ovanliga normalt. Kommunikativ varsamhet och medicinsk kontroll i barnmorskors samtal med gravida kvinnor* [Making the unusual normal: Communicative caution and medical control in talk between midwives and expectant mothers]. (Linköping Studies in Arts and Science No. 195). Linköping, Sweden: Department of Theme Research.

Bredmar, M., & Linell, P. (1999). Reconfirming normality: The constitution of reassurance in talks between midwives and expectant mothers. In S. Sarangi & C. Roberts (Eds.), *Talk, work and institutional order: Discourse in medical, mediation and management settings* (pp. 237–270). Berlin: Mouton de Gruyter.

Candlin, C., & Lucas, J. (1985). Interpretations and explanations in discourse: Modes of "advising" in family planning. In T. Ensink, A. van Essen, & T. van der Geest (Eds.), *Discourse analysis and public life* (pp. 13–38). Dordrecht, The Netherlands: Foris.

Candlin, S. (2002/this issue). Taking risks: An indicator of expertise? *Research on Language and Social Interaction, 35,* 173–193.

Cicourel, A. (1992). The interpenetration of communicative contexts: Examples from medical encounters. In A. Duranti & C. Goodwin (Eds.), *Rethinking context: Language as an interactive phenomenon* (pp. 291–310). Cambridge, England: Cambridge University Press.

Collins English Dictionary. (1991). (3rd ed.). Glasgow, Scotland: HarperCollins.

Douglas, M. (1992). *Risk and blame: Essays in cultural theory.* London: Routledge.

Giddens, A. (1991). *Modernity and self-identity.* Cambridge, England: Polity.

Hak, T. (1999). "Text" and "con-text": Talk bias in studies of health care work. In S. Sarangi & C. Roberts (Eds.), *Talk, work and institutional order: Discourse in medical, mediation and management settings* (pp. 427–451). Berlin: Mouton de Gruyter.

Harris, G. G. (1989). Mechanism and morality in patients' views of illness and injury. *Medical Anthropology Quarterly, 1,* 3–21.

Heritage, J. (2000). *Designing questions and setting agendas in the news interview.* Unpublished manuscript, University of California, Los Angeles.

Leppänen, V. (1998). *Structures of district nurse–patient interaction.* Lund, Sweden: Lund University, Department of Sociology.

Lindstedt, U. (1997). Att lotsa en patient genom en njurröntgen [Guiding a patient through a kidney X-ray]. *Master's thesis from tema K* (1997:4). Linköping, Sweden: Linköping University, Department of Communication Studies.

Linell, P. (1998). Discourse across boundaries: On recontextualizations and the blending of voices in professional discourse. *Text, 18,* 143–158.

Linell, P., & Bredmar, M. (1996). Reconstructing topical sensitivity: Aspects of face-work in talks between midwives and expectant mothers. *Research on Language and Social Interaction, 29,* 347–379.

Lupton, D. (1993). Risk as moral danger: The social and political functions of risk discourse in public health. *International Journal of Health Services, 23,* 425–435.

Peräkylä, A. (1997). Reliability and validity in research based on transcripts. In D. Silverman (Ed.), *Qualitative research: Theory, method and practice* (pp. 201–220). London: Sage.

Sachs, L., Taube, A., & Tishelman, C. (2001). Risk in numbers: Dilemmas in the transformation of genetic knowledge from research to people—the case of hereditary cancer. *Acta Oncologica, 4,* 445–453.

Sarangi, S., & Clarke, A. (2002/this issue). Zones of expertise and the management of uncertainty in genetics risk communication. *Research on Language and Social Interaction, 35,* 139–171.

Sarangi, S., & Roberts, C. (1999). The dynamics of interactional and institutional orders in work-related settings. In S. Sarangi & C. Roberts (Eds.), *Talk, work and institutional order: Discourse in medical, mediation and management settings* (pp. 1–57). Berlin: Mouton de Gruyter.

Silverman, D. (1997). *Discourses of counselling: HIV counselling as social interaction.* London: Sage.

Research on Language and Social Interaction, 35(2), 219–247

Agency and Authority: Extended Responses to Diagnostic Statements in Primary Care Encounters

Anssi Peräkylä
Department of Sociology and Social Psychology
University of Tampere

In this article, I explore patients' extended responses to doctors' diagnostic statements in Finnish primary care. As extended responses, I considered turns of talk that follow the doctors' diagnostic statements and in which the patients do something more than just acknowledge the diagnosis. The data consist of 71 diagnostic statements collected from a corpus of 100 video-recorded and transcribed general practice consultations. These data were analyzed using conversation analytic methods, both quantitative and qualitative. In the quantitative analysis, it was found that the patients produce extended responses after ⅓ of diagnostic statements. The type of the patient's response was found to be strongly associated with the way in which the doctor referred to the evidence for the diagnosis: After diagnostic statements in which the evidence is verbally explicated, the patients start to talk about the diagnosis more often than after diagnostic statements in which such explication is not done. In qualitative analysis, different types of extended responses were outlined. These include straight agreements, symptom descriptions, rejections of the proposed diagnoses, and actions related to the interpretation of evidence. In all types of extended responses, the patients displayed an orientation to the doctors' ultimate authority in the domain of medical reasoning.

In his seminal chapter, Heath (1992) showed that British patients regularly withhold responses to doctors' diagnostic statements, either by

Correspondence concerning this article should be sent to Anssi Peräkylä, Department of Sociology and Social Psychology, 33014 University of Tampere, Finland. E-mail: Anssi.Perakyla @uta.fi remaining completely silent or by producing just a minimal acknowledgment token such as a downward-intoned *er* or *yeh* after the doctor has told them the diagnosis. This passivity of patients in medical consultations is in contrast to the ways in which the recipients of news in ordinary conversation regularly and actively evaluate or mark as newsworthy the news that they are told (Maynard, 1997). Heath (1992) suggested that by withholding a response, the patients orient to a fundamental asymmetry between the doctors' knowledge and their own: They "relinquish or subordinate their knowledge and opinion concerning the illness and render the coparticipant's version as the objective, scientific, and factual assessment of the condition" (p. 264).

In this article, I explore Finnish patients' ways of responding to the doctors' diagnostic statements in the primary care environment. My main focus is on situations in which the patient responds more than minimally to the diagnosis. Extended responses occur after about one third of diagnostic statements. I explore different types of extended responses, showing how the participants cooperatively maintain a balance between the patients' agency and doctors' authority when such responses are given and received.

THE DOCTOR'S AUTHORITY AND THE PATIENT'S RESPONSE TO DIAGNOSIS

Authority is often considered a central quality of the doctor's relationship to the patient: The doctor is an expert who knows more (and is *entitled* to know more—see Drew, 1991) than the patient about the patient's possible illness (Abbott, 1988; Freidson, 1970; Parsons, 1951). Heath (1992) suggested that the doctor's authority as an expert is reproduced through the organization of interaction, among other things, in the practices through which the patients receive the diagnosis. In most cases in the British general practice consultations studied by Heath, the patients either remained silent or produced minimal acknowledgment tokens after the diagnosis. Through this kind of conduct, the patients treated the diagnosis as doctor's "property" and not as a relevant target for their own reflections.

However, in a few cases in Heath's British corpus, the patients did talk after the diagnosis. He (Heath, 1992) suggested that the patients' extended responses are associated with three features of diagnostic turns: Patient participation is encouraged by diagnoses (a) formatted as questions, (b) presented as uncertain, or (c) showing implicitly or explicitly that the doctor's view of the condition differs from what the patient expected (pp. 246–251; cf. Silverman, 1987, p. 48–85). In his analysis of the patients' extended responses, Heath (1992) focused on the asymmetry between the patients' "lay" views and the doctors' expert view. Open disagreements with the doctor are "extremely rare" (Heath, 1992, p. 258). At most, the patients resort to indirect and cautious utterances—involving, for example, descriptions of the subjective side of the illness—whereby they attempt to "encourage the doctor to reconsider the assessment of the complaint" (Heath, 1992, p. 258).

Authority and Accountability in the Delivery of Diagnosis

In a recent study, Peräkylä (1998) examined the ways in which Finnish primary care doctors display to their patients the evidence on which their diagnoses are based. Three designs of diagnostic utterances were identified: (a) in *plain assertions,* the doctors state the name of the illness in the classical proposition format "it is X," for example, by saying "that's already proper bronchitis"; (b) in diagnostic *turns incorporating inexplicit references to the evidence,* the doctor uses evidential verb constructions such as "it seems to be X," for example, by saying "no bacterial infection seems to be there"; (c) in *turns that explicate the evidence,* the doctor describes specific observations as evidence for the diagnostic statement, for example, by saying "as tapping on the vertebrae didn't cause any pain and there aren't yet any actual reflection symptoms in your legs it suggests a muscle complication."

The analytical upshot of Peräkylä's (1998) study was that in terms of the social relation between the patient and the doctor, there is something other than mere authority involved in the delivery of the diagnosis: It was argued that through the coordination of the design and placement of their diagnostic turns, the doctors treat themselves as *accountable* for the evidential basis of the diagnosis, thereby not claiming unconditional authority vis-à-vis the patients. These observations made it possible to qualify Parsons's (1951), Freidson's (1970), and Abbott's (1988) "absolutist" formulations concerning the doctors' authority: It was argued that instead of orienting themselves to the doctor's authority alone, the doctors and the patients maintain a specific *balance* between authority and accountability in the delivery of a diagnosis.

In this article, I continue this line of argumentation. Through the examination of the patients' extended responses to the doctor's diagnostic statements, I show that the patients in these situations assume a specific agency in the realm of diagnostic reasoning. This agency counterbalances the doctors' authority as an expert—just as the doctors' accountability for the evidential basis of their diagnoses does at an earlier stage of the diagnostic sequence. Thus, in this article, I explore the ways in which the participants maintain a specific balance between the patient's agency and the doctor's authority, in actions that follow the delivery of diagnosis.

Data and Methods

The method used in this research is conversation analysis (CA; Heritage, 1984b; Sacks, Schegloff, & Jefferson, 1974), and in particular CA as applied in the research on institutional interaction (Drew & Heritage, 1992). The CA approach has been used in research on medical interaction since the early 1980s (Frankel, 1983, 1984; Heath, 1984, 1986, 1989; West, 1984), and in recent years the number of CA studies in this field has been rapidly increasing (see, e.g., Heritage & Maynard, in press; Peräkylä, 1995; Ruusuvuori, 2001; Silverman, 1997). CA methodology usually entails a detailed case-by-case analysis of samples of interaction. In this article, however, the qualitative analysis is accompanied by a quantitative one (for quantitative applications of CA, see Heritage, 1995; Heritage & Roth, 1995).

More than 100 medical consultations in central Finland were video-recorded and transcribed. Four health centers (two serving residential areas and two large companies) were included in the data collection, and 14 doctors participated in the study. The number of consultations recorded per doctor varied. In each consultation recorded, the patient is different. Patients were not preselected according to their type of complaint or any other criteria.

From the recordings, all statements in which the doctor named the patient's illness were collected. Such statements were included only when the doctor named the illness for the first time either after the examination of the patient or after the patient had rejected an earlier diagnosis. Repeated diagnoses and prediagnostic "online commentary" (Heritage & Stivers, 1999) were excluded. This collection consists of 71 diagnostic statements occurring in 52 consultations. Each of the 14 doctors participating in the study gave at least one diagnostic statement. The highest number of diagnostic statements given by a doctor was 13; these statements were distributed across 10 different consultations. Quantitative analysis was used to identify the conditions in which patient's extended responses were likely to occur. The main analytical task, however, was qualitative, and it involved developing a typology of different types of extended responses to diagnostic statements and describing the interactional conditions and consequences of these practices.

The interactions presented in this article took place in the context of primary care. Practices of responding to diagnostic statements may be different in other types of medical contexts, such as specialized medicine or hospital medicine.

QUANTITATIVE ANALYSIS: WHEN IS THERE AN EXTENDED RESPONSE?

The patients' ways of receiving the doctors' diagnostic statements can be divided into three broad classes: (a) silence; (b) minimal acknowledgment tokens such as *yeah, yes,* and *ahem*[1]; and (c) extended responses. The last class includes all responses in which the patient does something more than just minimally acknowledge the diagnosis; for example, cases where they show that the diagnosis is "news" for them, or verbally indicate agreement or disagreement, or describe symptoms that may be discrepant with the diagnosis (for a closer description of these responses, see following).

In our sample of 71 diagnostic statements, these three types of responses are almost evenly distributed: No response was given by the patient in 23 cases, minimal acknowledgment was given in 25 cases, and an extended response was given in 23 cases. Thus, the Finnish patients actively took part in the diagnostic sequence in almost one third of cases and in one third they didn't. At least one extended response was produced in consultations of all except two doctors.

According to Heath (1992), active patient responses typically follow diagnoses that are formatted as questions, that are presented as uncertain, or that show implicitly or explicitly that the doctor's view of the condition differs from what the patient expected. In the Finnish data, there were no diagnoses formulated as questions. However, there were diagnoses that were presented as uncertain (e.g., by using probability markers) and those that showed discrepancy between the doctor's view and the patient's expectations. These features of diagnostic utterances are associated with the type of the patient's response also in the Finnish data (for details, see Peräkylä, in press). There was, however, also another stronger and statistically significant association (p = .001) between the type of the patient's response on one hand and the design of the doctor's diagnostic utterance on the other. More specifically, it was the way that the diagnostic utterance displayed evidence of the diagnostic conclusion that was associated with the type of response. Most of the extended responses occurred after diagnostic turns in which the doctor verbally explicated the evidence for the diagnostic conclusion. The two other diagnostic turn designs (turns incorporating inexplicit references to evidence and plain assertions with no reference to evidence) attracted far fewer extended responses. In particular, plain assertions were very infrequently followed by extended responses (see Table 1).

The explication of evidence makes it much more likely that the patient will produce an extended response to diagnosis than the two other diagnostic turn designs. Thus, it appears that by explicating the evidence for the diagnostic conclusion the doctor establishes a particular relation between the patient and himself or herself: one in which the patient's reflections on the diagnosis are relevant and welcome.[2]

Quantitative analysis of interaction remains, however, necessarily quite far from the actual dynamics of the momentarily unfolding actions of the people who are interacting (Schegloff, 1993). The distributional association between the design of the diagnostic turn on one hand and the pa-

TABLE 1
Diagnostic Turn Design and the Patient's Response

Diagnostic Turn Design	Patient's Response		
	None or Minimal	Extended	Total
Explication of evidence	12	16	28
Incorporated reference to evidence	9	3	12
Plain assertion	27	4	31
Total	48	23	71

Note. Pearson $\chi^2(2, N = XX) = 13.5079, p = .001$.

tients' inclination to respond on the other raise questions about the nature of the doctor's authority and the patient's agency in diagnostic sequences; but in dealing with these questions, I have thus far operated at a merely speculative level. To actually observe the construction of agency and authority in the diagnostic sequences, I have to resort to case-by-case analysis, which I present in the remaining parts of this article.

QUALITATIVE ANALYSIS: WHAT DO THE EXTENDED RESPONSES DO?

After one third of the diagnoses in our Finnish data, the patient does more than just acknowledge the diagnosis. In what follows, I present a qualitative analysis of these cases. The questions I address include the following: (a) What do the patients do in their extended responses to the diagnoses?, (b) what prompts the patients' responses in individual cases?, (c) how do the doctors treat the patients' responses?, and (d) how is the doctors' authority as an expert constructed in the context of the patients' responses? The discussion that follows is organized in terms of the first question: I proceed by exploring different types of actions that the patients may perform in their extended responses. In discussing these, I also address the other three questions.

Variety of Extended Responses

Patients' extended responses to diagnostic statements can take a wide variety of forms. I discuss the most regular forms in this article, but there are others, too, that I only mention. These less frequent forms of extended responses include, for example, *assessments* (Pomerantz, 1984; "It is, (0.6) it is quite a wonder," said after the doctor ruled out an illness) and *newsmarks* (Heritage, 1984a; Maynard, 1997; "Is there," said after the doctor told a patient that he has bronchitis). The diagnosis can also occasion *narration of the patient's earlier medical history* (i.e., storytelling about illnesses that were somehow comparable to the present one) and when the conclusion presented by the doctor is marked as uncertain *expressions of puzzlement.* However, as already indicated, all these forms of next actions after the diagnosis are infrequent, each represented by only one or two instances in the sample.

In what follows, I examine in detail some other types of extended next actions after the diagnosis. Taken together, these count as the majority of occasions of extended next actions in our sample. The next actions that I consider involve *straight agreements, symptom descriptions, alternative diagnosis proposals,* and *actions related to the interpretation of evidence.* These all are actions in which the patients in different ways take a stance to the very validity of the diagnosis that has been delivered by the doctor, thus treating themselves as agents capable of diagnostic reasoning. It is the patient's agency and its relation to the doctor's expertise that I am particularly interested in my analysis of data.

Straight agreements.   In some cases, the patients say that they agree with the diagnosis that the doctor has proffered. Extract 1[3] following is an example of this kind of situation (Dr. = doctor, P = patient):

(1) (Dgn 24 11B3)

```
 1   Dr:        Now there appears to be an (1.0) infection at the
 2              contact point of the joint below it in the sac of mucus
 3              there ⌈in the hip.   ⌉
 4   P:   →         ⌊Yes right. .hh ⌋that's what I(think)/(thought)
 5        →     myself too that <it probably must be an infection>.
 6              ⌈.hhhh
 7   Dr:        ⌊And, because you have had trouble this ⌈long we will
 8   P:                                                 ⌊hhhhh
 9   Dr:        make sure and take an X-⌈ray. ⌉
10   P:                                 ⌊Yes:.
```

The patient responds to a diagnostic statement in which the doctor indirectly referred to the inferential process by using the construction "appears to be." The diagnosis is also presented as uncertain. The doctor's diagnosis corresponds to one of the candidate explanations (Gill, 1998; Raevaara, 2000) offered by the patient during the examination. In lines 4 to 5, partially overlapping with the completion of the doctor's diagnostic statement, the patient responds with an acknowledgment and then expands her turn by saying "that's what I (think)/(thought) myself too that <it probably must be an infection>." (It is unclear whether the patient uses past or present tense of the verb *think.*) By reporting her agreement, the patient treats herself as an agent capable of diagnostic thinking. Yet in so doing, she also treats the realm of medical reasoning as something that ultimately belongs to the doctor. This is observable in a number of features.

First, the patient designs her agreement as arising from a distinct personal perspective. Through the turn beginning "that's what I thought myself too," she frames her agreement as a report of her own thoughts. She does not, like the doctor, describe objective realities but only reports her subjective perspective (Heath, 1992; Maynard, 1991). Second, the patient formulates the diagnosis using general terms ("it probably must be an infection"), thus portraying her conception of the illness as much more general than that of the doctor's, who had given a detailed specification concerning the site of the infection (in lines 1–2). Third, it is also noticeable that following the patient's turn, the doctor does not acknowledge, topicalize, or otherwise take note of the patient's report of her thoughts. Through the continuation marker "And" at the beginning of his turn in line 7, the doctor frames his talk about the further examinations as a continuation of the diagnostic statement (lines 1–3)—thus "sequentially deleting" the patient's comment. Through this nonattention, the doctor treats the diagnostic conclusion as not being a relevant target for the patient's comments.

In sum, therefore, in Extract 1 the patient assumed agency in diagnostic reasoning by expressing an explicit agreement with the doctor's diagnosis. This agency had both self-imposed and externally imposed limits: The patient presented her diagnostic thinking as markedly subjective and approximate, and the doctor treated the patient's statement as not a relevant target for further talk. Hence, along with allowing for the patient's agency, the participants collaboratively treated the details of the process of medical reasoning as something belonging exclusively to the doctor's domain.

Symptom descriptions. The most common type of patient's extended next action after the diagnosis is symptom description. Usually the postdiagnosis symptom descriptions display some kind of misalignment with the doctor's diagnosis. Consider Extract 2 following:

(2) (Dgn 38 40A2)

```
1  Dr:  H⌈as this< (0.6) f:oot of yours ever been x-rayed at
2  P:    ⌊( )( )
3  Dr:  °all°.
4  P:   °No::: (0.3) not ( ) ever.°
5       (1.2)
```

```
 6  P:    And then it really is: (.) it just is >>there ↑is such
 7        a bad °pain°.
 8        (0.5)
 9  Dr:   Yeah,
10  P:    ↑(  )
11  Dr:   You see this isn't a sciatica problem.
12        (0.3)
13  Dr:   .hh The problem is here m- (0.2) more in your ankle.
14  P:    Yes⌈::,
15  Dr:      ⌊only here in your ank⌈le.
16  P:                             ⌊Yeah, (.) .h and although it
17        also hurts if you sit in an armchair at home and get
18        up then it may (pinch) as far as here ac⌈tually.=here.
19  Dr:                                           ⌊(  )
20        (0.6)
21  Dr:   M⌈m:,
22  P:     ⌊(So) here.
23        (0.5)
24  P:    .mthh If the armchair is like somewhat awkward or
25        °something°.
26  Dr:   Yeah,
27  P:    °Mm° (hh)
28        (0.8)
29  Dr:   °°Yeah:,°°
30        (2.0)
31  Dr:   >So here<. .hhmt what we could do is to have an X-ray
32        of this (.hhh) (0.2) ankle of yours ((continues))
```

The patient has complained about a pain in her leg, and during the examination she suggests that it might be caused by the sciatic nerve (data not
shown). In lines 11 to 15, while the patient is still lying on the examination
table, the doctor gives a multiunit diagnostic statement. The statement involves an explicit conflict between the patient's expectations and the doctor's view. The doctor first (line 11) rejects the patient's earlier candidate
explanation (Gill, 1998; Raevaara, 2000), whereafter (in line 13) he as-
serts the location of the problem. Finally, in line 15, he renews and upgrades his assertion concerning the location.

After the first unit of the doctor's diagnostic statement, the patient remains silent. Following the second unit, she, in line 14, produces a neutral

response token, thereby acknowledging the doctor's assertion concerning the location of the ailment. The extended response takes place after the third unit in which the doctor renews and specifies his assertion. In line 16, the patient first acknowledges this assertion through "Yeah." After a micropause, she then goes ahead with a description of a location of pain. The beginning of her utterance ("Yeah, (.) .h and . . .") is designed in alignment with the doctor's preceding talk. However, as it unfolds, the patient's utterance turns out to be discrepant with the doctor's preceding assertion: She proposes that the pain occurs more widely than just in the ankle. The patient twice specifies the location of the pain through indexical "here," first as a direct continuation of her utterance in line 18 and then again in line 22 after a little gap and the doctor's neutral response token (line 21).

A gap ensues in line 23 after the patient has for a second time reasserted the location of the pain that she has been feeling. Uptake by the doctor would be possible here, as the patient's utterance is hearably completed (it has actually been recompleted twice). In absence of any action by the doctor, the patient however produces a further increment to her turn in lines 24 to 25. Now she adds a new "condition" to the appearance of the pain (it occurs with "awkward" armchairs).

Through this increment, the patient plays down the diagnostic relevancy of the symptom description that she has just given. The description was initially designed to be misaligned with the doctor's diagnosis. However, after the increment, the pain is no more portrayed as an anomaly requiring the doctor's attention but rather as something that has a "nonmedical," mundane cause (an awkward armchair). The patient played down the diagnostic relevancy of her symptom description in the face of no uptake by the doctor on the earlier parts of the description.

It is also noticeable that the doctor does not topicalize or otherwise take note of the patient's postdiagnosis symptom description, neither before nor after the reframing by the patient. In line 26 he produces a neutral acknowledgment token ("Yeah,"), and in line 29 he suggests the closure of the sequence through "Yeah:" said in *sotto voce*. Then, in line 31, he begins the announcement of future examinations.

In the preceding section of the article, I noted that conflict between the patient's and the doctor's views is, according to Heath (1992), one for features associated with the patients' inclination to respond to diagnosis. In Excerpt 2, the doctor's diagnostic utterance involved rejection of the patient's diagnostic proposal ("sciatica"). This rejection of her view may have put the patient on alert to respond. However, other local factors were at play, too.

The doctor's diagnosis was ambiguous in terms of its conclusiveness. The doctor asserted the *location* of the ailment, but did not yet name it. This assertion took place while the patient was still lying on the examination table, her body available for further examination. Therefore, the doctor's actions implied potential receptivity for further relevant information, and it is such information that the patient delivers in her response to the doctor's diagnostic utterance.

Extract 3 is another example of postdiagnostic symptom description that is designed to be discrepant with the diagnosis. The patient has complained about dizziness that began to occur after he had the flu. In the beginning of the physical examination, the doctor says that he will try and see whether an infection could be detected anywhere. In the beginning of the extract, he is examining the patient's sinuses using an ultrasound scan.

(3) (Dgn u7 - 35A4)

```
 1   Dr:   Small sinuses presumably because °it gives such a° low
 2         echo °(it gives).°
 3         (4.0)
 4   Dr:   (And) they have really the walls have got sturdier
 5         so,
 6         (0.4)
 7   Dr:   °Mhm.°
 8         (2.5)
 9   Dr:   °Here may even be some (real) disease°.
10         (0.5) ((Dr takes the scan away from P's face.))
11   P:    ⌈(((Sniffs))
12   Dr:   ⌊It gives from there (0.3) ech- (the) back wall
13         echo,
14         (1.0)
15   Dr:   from a few centimeters' depth so it does (.) mean
16         that they're (already) quite ↑full now,
17         (1.0) ((Dr gives a tissue to P))
18   Dr:   You can wipe your face with this.
19         (0.5)
20   Dr:   Presumably fuller than what you,
21         (1.0)
22   Dr:   otherwise have so h,
23         (0.5)
24   Dr:   That might actually somehow explain those symptoms
```

```
25         of yours.
26         (0.5)
27   P:    The thing is that there's actually been no
28         pai⌈n in them that there's no⌉thing (0.2) ⌈nothing's⌉ been
29   Dr:      ⌊(°Yeah°) mmm.          ⌋              ⌊.nfff  ⌋
30   P:    ⌈there.
31   Dr:   ⌊nyeah
32         (2.5)
33   Dr:   How sore the⌈se are.
34   P:                ⌊It does hurt when you do th⌈at.
35   Dr:                                           ⌊.hhh hhhehhh=
36   P:    =°(Well it ⌈does hurt°)⌉
37   Dr:              ⌊.hhhh      ⌋ (just) cause of the
38         dizziness of course in part if you feel that they
39         are like,
40         (0.5)
41   P:    Well when somebody presses you (.) ne⌈(h)xt t(h)o you(h)r
42   Dr:                                        ⌊hhhhhhhhh heh
43   P:    ea(h)r y(h)ou ⌈d(h)o f(h)eel⌉ p(h)ain .hhh=
44   Dr:                 ⌊heh heh      ⌋
45   Dr:   =.hh $Just put your shirt °on°.$
```

The doctor's diagnostic talk begins in line 9. At that point, however, he speaks in *sotto voce,* as if to himself while he is still scanning the patient's sinuses. This statement is, therefore, more like an "online commentary" (Heritage & Stivers, 1999) rather than a conclusive diagnosis. The diagnosis proper is delivered when the doctor resumes the diagnostic talk in line 12, after having completed the examination. He first explicates some of his observations concerning the "back wall echo," and thereafter, using the observations as evidence, in lines 15 to 16 he proffers a diagnostic conclusion "so it does (.) mean that they're (already) quite ↑full now." The doctor then gives the patient a tissue to wipe his face with and takes the scan to the other side of the room. When doing this (and while the patient is wiping his face), the doctor adds an increment to his diagnostic utterance (lines 20 and 22). Thereafter, in line 24, still expanding the same syntactical unit, he adds another part to the chain of inferences that he is laying out by proposing that what he has found could explain the patient's symptoms. This final part of the diagnostic utterance is also designed as uncertain.

During the first parts of the doctor's diagnostic statement, the patient remains silent (while he wipes his face). Only after having finished the wiping, in response to the doctor's proposal that what he has found could explain the patient's symptoms, the patient produces an extended turn of talk in lines 27 to 30. By reporting the absence of pain and other symptoms, he takes a stance toward the diagnosis: The "negative observations" are evidence against it. Thus, the patient assumes an active role in the realm of diagnostic reasoning.

In this case, unlike the one that I examined previously, the doctor does take notice of the patient's presentation of discrepant symptoms (or more specifically, of absence of symptoms). At first, his verbal uptake is minimal: The doctor gives acknowledgment tokens in lines 29 and 31. However, he addresses the issue of pain through another kind of action: When the patient is uttering his turn in line 28, the doctor begins to palpate the patient's head above his ears. In line 33 he then asks the patient to tell whether it hurts, and after the patient has answered in the affirmative, the doctor acknowledges the answer through a laugh token (line 35). The patient continues in humorous mode (lines 41 and 43). Through laughter and humor, both participants treat as noteworthy the fact that the doctor demonstrated pain in the patient's sinuses after the patient had claimed that there was none. By this demonstration, the doctor reestablished the validity of his diagnosis after the patient had reported absence of pain.

Extract 3 is, however, similar to the earlier one in one respect. Also here, the diagnostic statement that the patient responds to is ambiguous in terms of its conclusiveness. The first parts of the doctor's diagnostic talk that are addressed to the patient (lines 12–13, 15–16) are designed as conclusive. However, the part of the diagnosis that the patient actually responds to (line 24–25) is differently designed: In saying "That might actually somehow explain those symptoms of yours," the doctor moves to a more tentative mode and thereby creates a possible expectation of a more conclusive diagnosis to be achieved later. It is at this point that the patient produces his discrepant symptom description. Thus, again, it is possible that the patient produced his extended response in a situation in which he assumed the doctor's process of diagnostic reasoning to be not yet completed.

In describing symptoms that were discrepant with the diagnosis, the patients in Extracts 2 and 3 assumed agency in the realm of diagnostic reasoning: Instead of merely accepting the diagnosis, they told about something that was hearably in conflict with the diagnosis that the doctor had suggested. However, there were self-imposed limits to that agency as well. The patients did not address the diagnosis directly (by, e.g., rejecting it or expressing doubts about it), but they proffered their challenge in an indirect way by describing some of their experiences discrepant with the diagnosis. In Extract 3, in which the doctor described his observations as evidence for the diagnosis, the patient also did not topicalize the evidence or its relation to the diagnostic conclusion. Thus, the patients did not present a claim of agency in the discussion of diagnosis per se. The doctors, in receiving the patient's talk after diagnosis, operated in different ways, but in both cases they maintained their position as experts with authority. In Extract 2, the doctor first withheld even verbal acknowledgment of the patient's discrepant symptom description, proffering a full acknowledgment token only after the patient had backed down from the implicated diagnostic relevancy of her description. The acknowledgment did not lead to any further discussion: After it, the doctor continued to the next phase of the consultation (discussion on future action). In Extract 3, although the doctor did not verbally take up the patient's discrepant symptom description, he addressed it in direct physical means by demonstrating in a new phase of physical examination that what the patient had said was not the case.

Rejecting the diagnosis.   In cases discussed in the preceding section, the patients reported symptoms that were discrepant with the diagnosis given by the doctor. In those cases the patient's resistance toward the diagnosis was implied but not stated directly. However, in some other cases the patients do explicate their resistance, either by rejecting the doctor's diagnosis or by suggesting an alternative.

Consider Extract 4. Before the delivery of the diagnostic statement, the doctor has undertaken a long physical examination of the patient, who has complained about a sudden pain in her back. In lines 1 to 8, the doctor reports some of her observations while palpating the patient's back. She then withdraws from the patient (line 10), and while returning to her seat, she tells the patient her diagnostic conclusion. In her diagnostic utterance, the doctor first explicates the evidence for the diagnosis (lines 11–13), thereafter delivering the diagnosis proper (lines 13–14). Immediately after the diagnosis, she then moves on to speculate about the possible cause of the ailment (lines 14–15, 18–19).

(4) (Dgn 26 - 21A1)

```
1   Dr:   (But but) I really can feel these with my fingers
2         here it is you see ┌( ) this way, a very tight=
3   P:                       └Yes,
```

```
 4   Dr:   =muscle fibre,
 5         (1.0)
 6   P:    Yes a little th⌈ere<
 7   Dr:               ⌊IT GOes here from the top but
 8         it probably gives it (.) a bit further down then,
 9         (1.0)
10               ⌈((Dr withdraws her hands from P's back))
11   Dr:   As ⌊tapping on the vertebrae didn't cause any ↑pain
12         and there aren't (yet) any actual reflection
13         symptoms in your legs it corresponds with a
14         muscle h (.hhhh) complication so hhh it's⌈only
15         whether hhh (0.4) you                      ⌊
16                                             ⌊((Dr
17         lands on her chair.))
18         have been exposed to a draught or has it
19         otherwise=
20   P:    =Right,
21   Dr:   .Hh got irrita⌈ted,
22   P:                ⌊It couldn't be from somewhere
23         inside then as ↑it is a burning feeling there so
24         it couldn't be in the kidneys or somewhere (that
25         p⌈ain,)
26   Dr:   ⌊Have you had any tr- (0.2) trouble with
27         urinating.=
28         =a pa- need to urinate more frequently or
29         any pain when you urinate,
```

The patient's first response to the doctor's diagnostic statement occurs in line 20. Through her "Right," the patient receives the prior turn (concerning the possible origins of the ailment) as informative and as something that makes sense or can be agreed with, or both (cf. Heritage & Sefi, 1992; Sorjonen, 2001). The next time the patient speaks is in line 22, slightly overlapping with the completion of the doctor's reflections about the origin of the complication. The patient's comments are targeted at the diagnostic conclusion. Her utterance is constructed as a multiunit turn.

First, in line 22, the patient offers (in the form of a question) a characterization of the location of the trouble that (through its position and the marker "then") is marked as contrastive to what the doctor has said. Toward the end of her turn she specifies this location, again in the form of a yes–no question. In between these two proposals, she proffers evidence: "as ↑it is a burning feeling." Through the particle *as,* this symptom description is framed as evidence for the patient's diagnostic suggestions. Thus, this patient not only provides discrepant symptom description (which she does in line 23), but she also explicates her own diagnostic proposal concerning what these symptoms possibly could be a sign of (lines 22 and 24–25).

However, although assuming agency in the realm of medical reasoning, the patient also orients herself to the doctor's ultimate expertise and authority in the realm in which she is operating. Through the use of a question format in her diagnostic suggestions (lines 22–23 and 24–25) and through the question design that may prefer a negative answer to her suggestion, the patient displays a commitment that the doctor's view is correct and it is the doctor who will ultimately diagnose the trouble. The way in which she formulates her diagnostic proposals concerning the location of the ailment is nontechnical and approximate ("from somewhere inside then" and "in the kidneys or somewhere"). Moreover, the evidence that the patient produces in line 23 is of an "experiential" nature: By saying "as ↑it is a burning feeling," the patient describes a bodily sensation to which only she has access (cf. Peräkylä & Silverman, 1991). This subjective evidence is in contrast with the objective evidence produced by the doctor in lines 11 to 13 (cf. Maynard, 1991, p. 479).

In spite of their cautious and subjective character, the patient's diagnostic reflections are picked up by the doctor who, in lines 26 to 29, begins a verbal examination. The new examination (focusing on possible troubles with urinating) can be seen as motivated by the patient's suggestion that the trouble might reside in the kidneys. The doctor's questions follow immediately after the patient's query, and hence, they are offered as preliminary for answering the patient's question. In resuming the examination, the doctor acknowledges the patient's response as a legitimate basis for reconsidering the diagnosis. However, in so doing, she also acts as an expert whose ways of reasoning are different from those of the patient: She doesn't treat the "burning feeling" reported by the patient as a sufficient basis for *altering* the initial diagnosis but, instead, begins a doctor-driven collection of *new* potential evidence.

In addition to the fact that the patient's misalignment with the doctor's diagnosis is more explicit, there is also another feature that makes Extract 4 different from cases in which the patients produced mere symptom descriptions after the diagnostic statements. In Extract 4, the delivery of the doctor's diagnostic statement unequivocally marked the completion of the physical examination of the patient. At the very beginning of the diagnostic utterance (line 11), the doctor withdraws her hands from the patient's back. The core of the utterance is produced while she walks toward her chair, and the doctor lands on her chair in the beginning of the expansion of the diagnostic utterance in line 14. Thus, the examination is observably and accountably over when the doctor gives her diagnosis. The doctor has indicated that she is no longer seeking new information about the condition. The patient's selection of an action (Drew & Heritage, 1992) that questions the diagnosis directly rather than proffering a symptom description like the patients in Extracts 2 and 3 is alive to this: As the doctor has accountably closed the examination, new symptom information per se is not relevant any more, but instead, the patient must address the diagnostic conclusion more directly.[4]

Extract 5 is another example of a patient questioning the doctor's diagnosis. In this case, the patient has come for a health check. The extract is from the beginning of the consultation. The doctor is examining papers that may have come from a nurse who has seen the patient before the doctor.

(5) (Dgn 29 - 21A2)

```
 1   Dr:   So there's a hearing defect at some point hhhh
 2         (0.3) ((Dr goes through the papers))
 3   Dr:   ((Focusing her gaze on a paper:)) or well that
 4         doesn't actually look quite like a hearing defect
 5         that,
 6         (0.5) ((Dr gazes at the paper))
 7   P:    Mm::⌜::
 8   Dr:      ⌞cu:rve as there's such an even decline in the
 9         <other ear.>
10         (0.8) ((Dr gazes at the paper.))
11   P:    Well in a way probably a defect but it is
12         one tha::::t erm (0.4) has (.) appeared already
13         a long time ago an:d (2.0) I don't know then whether
14         it is:: from work or is i:t (.) from an illness
15         but (I don't),
16         (0.2)
17         B⌜ecause >you know I have< worked on a paper=
18   Dr:    ⌞Nyeah,
19   P:    =machine.
```

```
20   Dr:   Ye:┌:s,
21   P:        └In a paper factory,
22         (0.5)
23   Dr:   Ex┌actly,┐
24   P:      └So in┘ that sense: (0.2) it may be even from
25         that.
26         (0.3)
27   Dr:   .mhh
28         (0.5)
29   P:    Or not from that.
30   Dr:   Or not from that.
31         (0.3)
32   Dr:   When was it that this was first taken
33         notice of do you have any:
34         recollec┌tion: of r- that,        ┐
35   P:            └hh mmmm hhhhhhh┘
36         Might have been s:::a:y ten year┌s ago. hhhh┐h
37   Dr:                                    └'rs ago    ┘
38   Dr:   Yeah,=
39   P:    =Something was then:: (.) when the first curves
40         were taken then it was found that there is something
41         ((continues))
```

At line 1, the doctor names a prospective diagnosis (a hearing defect) that is likely found in the records. Subsequently, while looking at the actual hearing test result, she corrects herself (lines 3–5) and describes the evidence that she sees in the curve (lines 8–9). In his response to the diagnosis, the patient at first disagrees with the doctor's corrected diagnosis by insisting on the initial one: "Well in a way probably a defect" (line 11). He then proceeds to an elaborated account concerning the history and the background of the defect (lines 11–25). After the patient's account, the doctor takes up the patient's contrastive diagnostic proposal in her follow-up question that seeks more information about the history of the trouble (lines 32–34).

By insisting on a diagnosis that has been rejected by the doctor, the patient assumes a role in which he is capable of diagnostic thinking. However, the way in which he disagrees also betrays a constant orientation to the doctor's authority as an expert. Three features of the lengthy diagnostic segment are particularly significant. First, it is noticeable that the patient's disagreement is performed "in the auspices of" the doctor's initial diagnostic statement. It was the doctor who first said that there was a hearing defect, and thus, the patient insisted on a diagnosis that *the doctor* has first suggested, not a diagnosis that he himself would have independently arrived at. Second, in his account following the formulation of the disagreement, the patient draws not only on his own understanding but also on the expertise of other medical professionals. In lines 12 to 13, he tells the doctor that the alleged defect appeared a long time ago. By using a Finnish word, *ilmeni,* here, the patient suggests that the defect was identified by somebody other than himself, thus alluding to medical professionals who have been involved. The doctor hears the patient's talk this way, which is indicated by her choosing the passive form in her follow-up question in lines 32 to 33: She doesn't ask when the patient has taken notice of the problem, but rather when the problem "was first taken notice of," thus implicating the other person's possible involvement. Finally, in an expansion to his answer by referring to the time "when the first curves were taken" (lines 39–40), the patient unequivocally indicates the involvement of medical professionals (and medical technology) in the identification of the "defect." Third, when the patient moves on to speculate about the origin of the alleged defect, he suggests that it is caused by him having worked on a paper machine (lines 17–25). The doctor withholds uptake (see especially lines 26–28), and in the face of that, the patient explicitly backs down from his theory (line 29), thereby receiving marked acknowledgment from the doctor (line 30).

Thus, in Extract 5, in assuming agency in the realm of diagnostic reasoning, the patient simultaneously acknowledged the doctor's (and the medical profession's) expertise and authority in this area. The agency that he assumed was accountably produced by himself as agency operating in a world that is ultimately defined by the medical profession.

"Instructed seeing" of evidence.   As I pointed out in the first part of this article, the patients' expanded responses most often appear after diagnostic statements in which the doctors explicate the evidence of the diagnosis. Accordingly, most of the cases of expanded responses that I have examined in detail have followed such diagnostic statements. A feature that is common to all the cases examined thus far—and one that constitutes central evidence for the patients' orientation to the difference between their ways of reasoning and the doctors' ways of reasoning—needs to be reemphasized. It is the fact that in these cases, the patients systemati-

cally did not refer to, contest, or otherwise talk about the evidence that the doctors were using.

Thus, in Extract 3, the patient who produced a discrepant symptom description after the diagnosis concerning sinuses in no way questioned the doctor's assertion that the "back wall echo" comes from a few centimeters' depth, that this is evidence for the sinuses being "quite full," and that this in turn could explain his dizziness. Also, in Extract 4, the patient who produced her alternative diagnostic proposal did not question whether "no pain in vertebrae" or "no reflection symptoms in legs" are valid evidence for her problem involving a muscle complication. Yet again, in Extract 5, the patient who openly insisted on a diagnosis that had been rejected by the doctor did not call into question, or in any way refer to, the shape of the curve that the doctor presented as evidence for her diagnosis that there was no hearing defect. By leaving "intact" the evidence that the doctors were displaying, these patients (who directly or indirectly misaligned with the diagnosis) treated the doctors' ways of reasoning and their own ways of reasoning as different, as operating on different domains as it were.

However, there are a small number of cases in which the patients do take up the evidence presented by the doctors. In this last empirical section of the article, I discuss two such cases. I show that even when taking up the doctor's evidence, the patients and the doctors orient to a fundamental difference in their respective ways of reasoning.

Consider Extract 6. This is an example of a relatively rare (but nonetheless existent) practice of a doctor showing to the patient the medical document that the diagnosis is based on. The patient is a building worker who has come for a health check. The doctor has identified a hearing defect.

(6) (Dgn U19 - 32B1)

```
 1   Dr:   Then the ↑other ones were taken,
 2         (0.2)
 3   ?:    °.hhh°
 4         (0.9) ((Doctor shuffles papers.))
 5   Dr:   Hearing and si:ght,
 6         (0.5) ((The doctor places a paper between himself and
 7         the patient))
 8   Dr:   And here you see really in this hearing curve that in
 9         your right ear the hearing faculty drops a little so
10         if you compare it to this earlier curve so °erm°
```

```
11        you'll see that °hh it has come ↑down a °little°. (.)
12   P:   So it seems to have °done°,
13   ?Dr: °Yeah:°,
14        (.)
15   Dr:  And this is of >the< noise damage type so that it
16        drops here then below this· black line to this side so
17        it then drops down °probably°,
          ((14 lines of further explanation dropped))
32   Dr:  °.Hhh° but this is not to be worried about however
33        >your left ear< is quite good >but there's also< some
34        beginning of a hollow already.
35   Dr:  ((Beginning to move the paper aside:)) tch so this
36        >is now< (.) a question of hearing protection more or
37        less so,
38   ?P:  °.Hhhh°
39        (0.3) ((Dr is shuffling the papers.))
40   ?P:  °Ehhhh hhhh°
41   Dr:  °So° how active have you been in hearing protection
42        I mean is it °hhh°
```

In line 8, the doctor begins a diagnostic statement. He has previously picked up a paper with the hearing test results and placed it on the desk between himself and the patient; the paper remains on the table until line 35, when the doctor moves it away. As long as the paper is on the table, the doctor, while speaking, points to the curve with a pen, and the patient looks at the paper. The doctor invites the patient to take part in seeing and interpreting the curve by verbally formulating the *patient's* perception in lines 8 to 11 ("here you see"; "if you compare"; "you'll see"). Throughout the segment, he uses pronominal constructions that presuppose that the patient sees the same as the doctor. Major parts of the segment are then designed as *instructions for seeing:* The doctor shows to the patient different parts of the curve, simultaneously interpreting their meaning (cf. Goodwin, 1994).

The patient's verbal response to the diagnosis occurs after the first upshot of the diagnostic statement in line 12. By saying "So it seems to have done," the patient confirms that the new curve has "come down"; by using the evidential "seems," he also confirms that he sees what the doctor has shown to him. Now, as it was pointed out previously, this patient comes further than most of the others into the territory usually occupied by doctors: Unlike the others, he takes part in the interpretation *of the same evidence* that the doctor accountably is using as the basis of his diagnosis. By the same token, it is clear that the patient's agency in the interpretation of this evidence is of reactive character: The doctor *invites* the patient to look at the evidence, he *shows* him the relevant parts of the evidence, and he *instructs* him in seeing them in the correct way. Thus, when the patient formulates "his" interpretation of the evidence in line 12, he merely confirms that he sees what the doctor has shown to him. All this amounts to the fact that the doctor's authority as an expert in interpreting the evidence is collaboratively upheld by both parties *at the same time* as the evidence of the diagnosis is made available for the patient's scrutiny.

Extract 7 is a parallel case. The patient has come for a checkup for her damaged wrist, which has been put in a plaster. Somewhat earlier in this consultation, the doctor has examined new X-rays of the wrist and has told the patient that the position of the bones has remained good. After some intervening talk, in the beginning of the extract, the doctor moves to announce the length of the time that the patient needs to wear the plaster cast. The announcement is met by the patient's display of surprise (lines 3 and 6), leading the doctor to account for the time in lines 5 and 9 to 10. As an expansion to this sequence, the patient, in lines 15 to 16, asks the doctor to confirm that there is no problem in the X-rays. (The doctor has picked up the X-rays anew from the table, and in line 13 he possibly glances at them.)

(7) (Dgn 60 - 40A1)

```
 1   Dr:   And well (.) it's five weeks: tha:t (.) usually I think
 2         the plaster cast is wo⌈rn °(so)°.⌉
 3   P:                          ⌊I see, it's⌋ as long as that.
 4         (.)
 5   Dr:   ⌈Well, that's wha:t I have last,     ⌉
 6   P:    ⌊Oh gosh (there's) no ah hah haa⌋
 7         (0.5)
 8   P:    Mm::::,
 9   Dr:   hear- (.) heard about so that's what is
10         ↓recommended.
11         (y⌈eah).
12   P:      ⌊Yeah.
13   Dr:   .thh (.) Yes,
14         (.)
15   P:    ((Leaning toward the X-rays:)) So no problem then
```

```
16        so: it ⌈is, (.) so one can't see t⌈here in them,
17   Dr:      ⌊(Yeah)<                    ⌊(m-)
18   Dr:   Yes:. Here you can look ⌈yours-⌉
19   P:                            ⌊Yeah, ⌋ I
20        ⌈saw them the⌉ first x-rays ⌈then.              ⌉
21   Dr:  ⌊yourself so, ⌋              ⌊ and compare th⌋ at to
22        this other one so it's quite in the same ⌈position.
23   P:                                             ⌊So it
24        seems to be yes.
25   Dr:  ⌈Might be⌉ even: (0.5) even somehow little
26   P:   ⌊Yes.   ⌋
27   Dr:  impro⌈ved     ⌉ that p⌈osition actually.
28   P:        ⌊Improv-⌋       ⌊Yeah:.
29   P:   °Yeah°.
```

Unlike in Extract 6, here the patient takes the initiative to see the X-rays. In line 15, when eliciting the doctor's reconfirmation concerning the "no problem" status of her hand, the patient leans toward the X-ray pictures that are in the doctor's hand, thereby indicating her willingness to see them. She also formulates the last part of her question ("so one can't see there in them") in a way that refers to the X-ray pictures. Thus, the patient is here questioning the "no problem" diagnosis that the doctor delivered earlier, and in doing so she also searches for access to the evidence that the doctor was using in delivering the diagnosis.

In his answer to the patient's question, the doctor gives the reconfirmation through "Yes:." (line 18; cf. line 17). Immediately after the reconfirmation, he proceeds to offer the evidence for the patient to see; the verbal offer in line 18 is accompanied by a movement in which the doctor lifts up the X-rays toward the light coming from the window, in a position where the patient can see them. Instructions for seeing (comparable to those in Extract 6) follow in lines 21 to 22, and in lines 23 to 24, the patient confirms that she sees what the doctor was instructing her to see, again using the evidential "seems," similar to the patient in Extract 6. In lines 25 and 27, the doctor upgrades his interpretation of the X-rays, still holding the pictures up for him and the patient to see, until the last word of line 27 in which he brings down the X-rays. The patient confirms, now using partial repeat (line 28) and agreement tokens (lines 28 and 29). Thus, in Extract 7, it was the patient who took the initiative in asking for access to the evidential documents that formed the basis of the diagnosis; however, when interpreting the documents, the patient was as reactive as the one in Extract 6, confining her role to the acknowledgment of what the doctor instructed her to see.

CONCLUSIONS

In this article, I have explored the patients' extended responses to the doctors' diagnostic statements. I started by noting that the Finnish primary care patients respond with more than acknowledgment tokens after about one third of doctors' diagnostic statements. Comparable exact numbers of patient responses have not been provided in earlier research, but the thrust of Heath's (1992) influential discussion suggests that the British patients in the 1980s may have been more passive than the Finnish patients in the 1990s.

In the quantitative part of this study, I also found that the extended responses are most likely to occur after diagnostic statements in which the doctors explicate the evidence for the diagnostic conclusion. This observation has direct practical implications: It suggests that if (in a particular consultation) the doctor welcomes the patient's participation in discussion about diagnosis, one thing that doctor can do to foster such participation is to indicate to the patient some of the evidential grounds of the diagnosis.

In the qualitative analysis, I deepened my understanding of the patient's extended responses. I characterized some of the actions that the patients perform in their responses: Straight agreements, symptom descriptions, alternative diagnosis proposals, and actions related to the interpretation of evidence were among them. My exploration of individual cases deepened my understanding of these actions in two respects: (a) in terms of the relation between the patients' responses and the other activities performed in the medical consultation and (b) in terms of the management of agency and authority in these consultations.

Patients' responses and other activities in consultations.   The qualitative analysis showed how the patients' extended responses are fitted to the local contingencies of their occurrence. I suggested that the conclusiveness of the diagnosis is central here. If the diagnostic utterance is positioned before a marked closure of examination (cf. Heritage & Stivers, 1999), or if it is designed as preliminary or partial, it may suggest to the patient that the diagnostic process may not yet be closed and a symptom description by the patient may be due. On the other hand, when the examination was markedly closed in conjunction with the diagnosis, the patients' responses addressed directly the diagnostic conclusion.

The management of the patient's agency and the doctor's expertise. In terms of the epistemic relations between the participants, the fact that the patients are passive after diagnosis in two thirds of the cases remains a primary indication of their submission in the face of medical authority, just as Heath (1992) suggested. By remaining passive, the patients can also indicate their expectation that discussion on treatment or other future action is due after the delivery of diagnosis (cf. Robinson, 2000). However, my primary interests here were the one third of the cases in which the patients responded actively. I noted (again, essentially in line with Heath's [1992] earlier observations) that the patients design these responses in a cautious manner, consistently displaying an orientation to the difference between their own and the doctors' ways of reasoning. The primary way for the patients to express their reservations toward the diagnosis is to offer additional observations (usually symptom descriptions) discrepant with the diagnosis. These additional observations come from outside the realm of the physical examination or the examination of documents: They are not observations of the things that the doctor has been examining, but they are about something that the patient has direct access to (bodily sensations or reports from everyday life). If the doctors present their observations as evidence to support the diagnosis, the patients in most cases systematically refrain from any discussion concerning these observations, let alone from questioning the inferential procedures from the observations to the diagnostic conclusion. Also, in the few cases in which the doctor's observations are addressed by the patients, they adopt a reactive and dependent position in the interpretation of this evidence.

I also saw that the doctors' ways of dealing with the patients' responses vary from virtual inattention (sequential deletion) to uptake through return to medical interview and physical examination; but in each way of dealing with the patients' response, the doctors also maintained their status as experts in the realm of medical reasoning.

In conclusion, the extracts of extended responses that I have examined suggest that primary care patients can, and in a number of cases do, assume a measure of agency in relation to their diagnoses. They have available ways for displaying agreement and disagreement with the diagnosis. However, this agency is intertwined and also overshadowed by the patients' and the doctors' orientation to the doctor's expertise and authority in the realm of medical reasoning. This dual orientation is perhaps most strikingly encapsulated in those cases in which the patient responds to diagnostic utterances in which the doctor has explicated the evidence for his or her conclusion (and that is where most of the active responses occur). The explication of evidence indirectly suggests that it is relevant also for the patients to talk after the diagnosis. However, in their talk that follows the diagnosis, the patients systematically avoid addressing the very evidence that the doctors explicated.

NOTES

1   These are English representations of Finnish response tokens used in the consultations. The original Finnish tokens include, for example, *Joo., Juu., Nii., Jaa::, Mm:* and *Aha* (cf. Sorjonen, 2001). Some of the minimal acknowledgment tokens are designed to encourage further elaboration of the diagnostic statement or its implications in terms of treatment, whereas others do not overtly have such characteristics. Silences may also operate as elicitation of elaboration (cf. Maynard, 1997). Further research is evidently needed regarding the work that the minimal responses and silences do after the diagnostic statements (see Robinson, 2000, for a discussion on "progressivity" between the diagnostic sequence and the talk about diagnosis).

2   As shown in an earlier article (Peräkylä, 1998), explication of evidence is a practice that doctors often resort to when the diagnosis is uncertain or involves conflict. Thus, the explication of evidence is a reflexive practice through which the doctors can *retrospectively* treat the diagnostic procedure as having involved some problem and *prospectively* make relevant the patient's participation in it.

3   The original Finnish transcripts and word-by-word translations are available from Anssi Peräkylä.

4   Consider also Extract 1 in which the patient also addressed the diagnosis directly but in agreement with the doctor. Also in that case, the doctor had accountably and observably completed the examination (after the completion of the examination but prior to the diagnostic statement, he was working with a computer preparing a referral to X-ray).

REFERENCES

Abbott, A. (1988). *The system of professions: An essay on the division of expert labor.* Chicago: The University of Chicago Press.

Drew, P. (1991). Asymmetries of knowledge in conversational interactions. In I. Markova & K. Foppa (Eds.), *Asymmetries in dialogue* (pp. 29–48). Hemel Hempstead, England: Harvester Wheatsheaf.

Drew, P., & Heritage, J. (1992). Analyzing talk at work: An introduction. In P. Drew & J. Heritage (Eds.), *Talk at work* (pp. 3–65). Cambridge, England: Cambridge University Press.

Frankel, R. (1983). The laying on of hands: Aspects of the organization of gaze, touch and talk in the medical encounter. In S. Fisher & A. D. Todd (Eds.), *The social organization of doctor–patient communication* (pp. 19–54). Washington, DC: Center for Applied Linguistics.

Frankel, R. (1984). From sentence to sequence: Understanding the medical encounter through microinteractional analysis. *Discourse Processes, 7,* 135–170.

Freidson, E. (1970). *Professional dominance.* Chicago: Aldine.

Gill, V. (1998). Doing attributions in medical interactions: Patients' explanations for illness and doctors' responses. *Social Psychology Quarterly, 61,* 342–360.

Goodwin, C. (1994). Professional vision. *American Anthropologist, 96,* 606–633.

Heath, C. (1984). Talk and recipiency: Sequential organization in speech and body movement. In J. M. Atkinson & J. Heritage (Eds.), *Structures of social action* (pp. 247–265). Cambridge, England: Cambridge University Press.

Heath, C. (1986). *Body movement and speech in medical interaction.* Cambridge, England: Cambridge University Press.

Heath, C. (1989). Pain talk: The expression of suffering in the medical consultation. *Social Psychology Quarterly, 52,* 113–125.

Heath, C. (1992). The delivery and reception of diagnosis and assessment in the general practice consultation. In P. Drew & J. Heritage (Eds.), *Talk at work* (pp. 235–267). Cambridge, England: Cambridge University Press.

Heritage, J. (1984a). A change-of-state token and aspects of its sequential placement. In J. M. Atkinson & J. Heritage (Eds.), *Structures of social action* (pp. 299–345). Cambridge, England: Cambridge University Press.

Heritage, J. (1984b). *Garfinkel and ethnomethodology.* Cambridge, England: Polity.

Heritage, J. (1995). Conversation analysis: Methodological aspects. In U. M. Quasthoff (Ed.), *Aspects of oral communication* (pp. 391–418). Berlin: de Gruyter.

Heritage, J., & Maynard, D. W. (in press). Introduction: Analyzing interaction between doctors and patients in primary care encounters. In J. Heritage & D. W. Maynard (Eds.), *Practicing medicine: Structure and process in primary care encounters.* Cambridge, England: Cambridge University Press.

Heritage, J., & Roth, A. (1995). Grammar and institution: Questions and questioning in the broadcast news interview. *Research on Language and Social Interaction, 28,* 1–60.

Heritage, J., & Sefi, S. (1992). Dilemmas of advice: Aspects of the delivery and reception of advice in interactions between health visitors and first time mothers. In P. Drew & J. Heritage (Eds.), *Talk at work* (pp. 359–417). Cambridge, England: Cambridge University Press.

Heritage, J., & Stivers, T. (1999). Physicians' on-line commentary: A method of modifying patients' diagnostic expectations. *Social Science and Medicine, 49,* 1501–1517.

Maynard, D. W. (1991). Interaction and institutional asymmetry in clinical discourse. *American Journal of Sociology, 97,* 448–495.

Maynard, D. W. (1997). The news delivery sequence: Bad news and good news in conversational interaction. *Research on Language and Social Interaction, 30,* 93–130.

Parsons, T. (1951). *The social system.* New York: Free Press.

Peräkylä, A. (1995). *AIDS counselling: Institutional interaction and clinical practice.* Cambridge, England: Cambridge University Press.

Peräkylä, A. (1998). Authority and accountability: The delivery of diagnosis in primary health care. *Social Psychology Quarterly, 61,* 301–320.

Peräkylä, A. (in press). Communicating and responding to diagnosis. In J. Heritage & D. Maynard (Eds.), *Practicing medicine: Structure and process in primary care encounters.* Cambridge, England: Cambridge University Press.

Peräkylä, A., & Silverman, D. (1991). Owning experience: Describing the experience of other persons. *Text, 11,* 441–480.

Pomerantz, A. (1984). Agreeing and disagreeing with assessments: Some features of preferred/dispreferred turn shapes. In J. M. Atkinson & J. Heritage (Eds.), *Structures of social action* (pp. 57–101). Cambridge, England: Cambridge University Press.

Raevaara, L. (2000). *Potilaan diagnoosiehdotukset lääkärin vastaanotolla. Keskustelunanalyyttinen tutkimus potilaan institutionaalisista tehtävistä* [Patients' diagnostic suggestions in primary care consultations: Conversation analytic study of patients' institutional tasks]. Helsinki, Finland: Suomalaisen Kirjallisuuden Seura.

Robinson, J. (2000). *The organization of action and activity in general practice doctor–patient consultations.* Unpublished doctoral dissertation, University of California, Los Angeles.

Ruusuvuori, J. (2001). Looking means listening: Coordinating displays of engagement in doctor–patient interaction. *Social Science and Medicine, 52,* 1093–1108.

Sacks, H., Schegloff, E. A., & Jefferson, G. (1974). A simplest systematics for the organization of turn-taking for conversation. *Language, 50,* 696–735.

Schegloff, E. A. (1993). Reflections on quantification in the study of conversation. *Research on Language and Social Interaction, 26,* 99–128.

Silverman, D. (1987). *Communication and medical practice: Social relations in the clinic.* London: Sage.

Silverman, D. (1997). *Discourses of counselling: HIV counselling as social interaction.* London: Sage.

Sorjonen, M.-L. (2001). *Responding in conversation. A study of response particles in Finnish.* Amsterdam: Benjamins.

West, C. (1984). *Routine complications: Troubles with talk between doctors and patients.* Bloomington: Indiana University Press.

SUBSCRIPTION ORDER FORM

Please ❑ enter ❑ renew my subscription to:

RESEARCH ON LANGUAGE AND SOCIAL INTERACTION

Volume 35, 2002, Quarterly — ISSN 0835–1813/E-ISSN 1532–7973

SUBSCRIPTION PRICES PER VOLUME:

Individual:
❑ $40.00 US/Canada
❑ $70.00 All Other Countries

Institution:
❑ $345.00 US/Canada
❑ $375.00 All Other Countries

Electronic Only:
❑ $36.00 Individual
❑ $310.50 Institution

Subscriptions are entered on a calendar-year basis only and must be paid in advance in U.S. currency—check, credit card, or money order. Prices for subscriptions include postage and handling. Journal prices expire 12/31/02. NOTE: Institutions must pay institutional rates. Individual subscription orders are welcome if prepaid by credit card or personal check. Electronic access is available at no additional cost to full-price print subscribers. Electronic-only subscriptions are available at a reduced price.

❑   Check Enclosed (U.S. Currency Only)   Total Amount Enclosed $_____

❑   Charge My: ❑ VISA   ❑ MasterCard   ❑ AMEX   ❑ Discover

Card Number _____   Exp. Date_____/_____

Signature_____
(Credit card orders cannot be processed without your signature.)

PRINT CLEARLY for proper delivery. STREET ADDRESS/SUITE/ROOM # REQUIRED FOR DELIVERY.

Name_____

Address_____

City/State/ Zip+4 _____

Daytime Phone #_____E-mail address_____
Prices are subject to change without notice.

Please note: A $20.00 penalty will be charged against customers providing checks that must be returned for payment. This assessment will be made only in instances when problems in collecting funds are directly attributable to customer error.

For information about online subscriptions, visit our website at *www.erlbaum.com*

Mail orders to: **Lawrence Erlbaum Associates, Inc.,** Journal Subscription Department
10 Industrial Avenue, Mahwah, NJ 07430; (201) 236–9500; FAX (201) 760–3735

LIBRARY RECOMMENDATION FORM

Detach and forward to your librarian.

❑ I have reviewed the description of *Research on Language and Social Interaction* and would like to recommend it for acquisition.

RESEARCH ON LANGUAGE AND SOCIAL INTERACTION

Volume 35, 2002, Quarterly — ISSN 0835–1813/E-ISSN 1532–7973

Institutional Rate: ❑ **$345.00** (US & Canada)   ❑ **$375.00** (All Other Countries)

Name_____Title_____

Institution/Department_____

Street Address_____

Signature_____Date_____/_____/_____
Librarians, please send your orders directly to LEA or contact from your subscription agent.

Lawrence Erlbaum Associates, Inc., Journal Subscription Department
10 Industrial Avenue, Mahwah, NJ 07430; (201) 236–9500; FAX (201) 760–3735

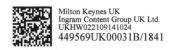